THE ABORTION DEBATE IN THE WORLD ARENA

The Abortion Debate in the World Arena

Andrzej Kulczycki

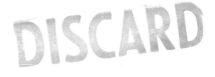

Routledge
New York

Published in 1999 by
ROUTLEDGE
29 West 35th Street
New York, NY 10001

Library of Congress Cataloging-in-Publication Data
Kulczycki, Andrzej
   The abortion debate in the world arena / by Andrzej Kulczycki.
      p.   cm.
   Includes bibliographical references and index.
   ISBN 0–415–92267–4 (hb). — ISBN 0–415–92268–2 (pb)
   1. Abortion—Moral and ethical aspects.   2. Abortion—Cross
   -cultural studies.   I. Title.
   HQ767.15.K86   1999
   363.46—dc21   98–11649
                                                                     CIP

This book is printed on paper suitable for recycling and made from fully managed and sustained forest sources.

Printed in Great Britain

To Lucía

the wonderful woman in my life

Contents

List of Tables and Figures

Tables

Figures

List of Abbreviations

AIDS	acquired immunodeficiency syndrome
CELAM	Latin American Episcopal Conference (Conferencia Episcopal Latinoamericana)
CFFC	Catholics for a Free Choice
CONAPO	National Population Council (Consejo Nacional de Población) (Mexico)
D&C	dilatation and curettage
FIGO	International Federation of Gynecology and Obstetrics
FLCAK	Family Life Counselling Association of Kenya
FPAK	Family Planning Association of Kenya
GIRE	Reproductive Rights Information Group (Grupo de Información en Reproducción Elegida)
IMSS	Mexican Social Security Institute (Instituto Mexicano de Seguro Social)
IPAS	International Projects Assistance Services
IPPF	International Planned Parenthood Federation
IUD	intrauterine device
IVF	in-vitro fertilization
KANU	Kenya African National Union
KCS	Kenya Catholic Secretariat
KDHS	Kenya Demographic and Health Survey
KMA	Kenya Medical Association
MCH	maternal and child health
MEXFAM	Mexican Foundation for Family Planning (Fundación Mexicana Para la Planificación Familiar)
MOH	Ministry of Health
MVA	manual vacuum aspiration
NAFTA	North American Free Trade Agreement
NCCK	National Council of Churches of Kenya
NCPD	National Council for Population and Development (Kenya)
NFP	natural family planning
NGO	non-governmental organization
PAN	National Action Party (Partido de Acción Nacional) (Mexico)
PRI	Institutional Revolutionary Party (Partido Revolucionario Institucional) (Mexico)

Abbreviations

SLD	Democratic Left Alliance (Sojusz Lewicy Demokratycznej)
STD	sexually transmitted disease
TFR	total fertility rate
UN	United Nations
UNDP	United Nations Development Programme
UNEP	United Nations Environment Programme
UNICEF	United Nations Children's Fund
UNFPA	United Nations Population Fund (formerly known as the United Nations Fund for Population Activities)
USA	United States of America
USAID	United States Agency for International Development
WHO	World Health Organization
ZChN	Christian National Union (Zjednoczenie Chrześcijańskie Narodowe)

Preface

One morning in Nairobi a soft-spoken man told me how he came across a small bundle by some rocks near a river. He looked more closely and recoiled when he saw a dead infant. The women in the makeshift houses nearby said the young mother had come from a broken home; their only surprise was that she had given birth and had not aborted her pregnancy. 'One cannot fix a social problem with a medical solution,' continued the person, a compassionate religious figure. The encounter prompted him to help set up a counselling center for disadvantaged women with crisis pregnancies which also intervened on behalf of pregnant girls to let them return to school and complete their education.

That same day I met an earnest physician who told a different story about two schoolgirls who became pregnant at a summer camp. One of the girls had a father willing and able to pay for an abortion. The other girl did not. Expelled from school, she attempted to stay with her uncle, who disowned her. After she gave birth at a public hospital, she could only afford slum housing and did what she could to make ends meet. Fifteen years later and looking prematurely aged, the woman was brought to court for brewing and selling illicit alcohol. There she met her old classmate, now her judge. 'What was the one single event that caused the change in fortunes and parting of the ways?', the physician asked.

These stories suggest some of the human dimensions to the problems posed by unwanted pregnancies and abortions, the deep concern this evinces among many people, and how individual decisions about abortions are made often as if on a separate plane from that where public debate about abortion takes place. In fact, most of the 45–50 million annual abortions worldwide are thought to be operated on women in more stable relationships than in the stories above; women who already have children and who for various reasons feel they cannot bear more. They are rarely willing to discuss their experiences, reflecting a moral, emotional and social complexity seldom apparent in public debates about abortion. And yet the way this issue is resolved in the public arena will in large part determine how abortion is thought of and the way in which it is likely to occur.

Abortion is perhaps the oldest method of controlling fertility, and it remains a health problem in many societies; over 150 women die each day due to their pregnancies being terminated under unsafe conditions. Abortion touches deep questions about values and brings up primordial sentiments. It is tied to the broad sphere of sexuality and reproductive life that many people find awkward to discuss. It cuts across gender, social, religious and political cleavages.

Arguments about abortion, and the question of what to do about it, are no longer confined to the Western liberal democracies. Understanding the dynamics of the abortion debate has become a vital area for comparative international research. The US government, feminist forces and the Holy See waged a highly publicized battle over abortion before and during the 1994 UN International Conference on Population and Development, held in Cairo. The European Union, Latin American states and Islamic governments also became involved in this bitter dispute that dominated the conference proceedings and received global media coverage, graphically illustrating the arrival of the abortion issue on the international agenda.

This book attempts to compare, contrast and link the abortion debate globally by using multiple sources of evidence, including 162 elite interviews. The study shows how and why controversy over abortion has spilled over to the developing world and to the postcommunist societies of East Central Europe. This assessment is enhanced by being empirically grounded in the experiences of three nations – Kenya, Mexico and Poland. These countries, often considered as regional bellwethers, are strategically significant in the worldwide struggle between groups over abortion. In each of these countries, domestic processes and international influences are focusing greater attention on abortion. These forces include organized Catholicism and women's movements. Abortion is being discussed more openly than before, and its practice is most unlikely to decline unless contraceptive use becomes more widespread and effective.

The complexity of the abortion debate involves historical and cultural meanings specific to each country. It also reflects different stages of demographic transition and reliance on abortion for fertility regulation, as well as struggles over gender roles, laws, relations between church and state, the influence of other social actors, and the way the policymaking system works. Consideration of such variance facilitates comprehension of cross-national similarities and differences in the social construction of abortion, its management and the conflict surrounding it. The ensuing debate is often poorly informed at the same time as it is moving to the public arena, be it slowly as in Kenya and Mexico, or more rapidly as in Poland. It is reaching agenda status as societies become more pluralistic and open to external interests, and states are finding it more difficult to contain the controversy and to reach an effective policy resolution.

The Abortion Debate in the World Arena consists of five chapters. Chapter 1 outlines the key dimensions to 'the policy conundrum' posed by abortion, the scope and purpose of the study, the issues and themes with which it is concerned, as well as the reasons for looking at Kenya, Mexico and Poland in more depth. The methodology is discussed further in an appendix. Chapters 2, 3 and 4 examine abortion practice, policy and debate in Kenya, Mexico and Poland, respectively, and address a range of shared underlying concerns with a focus on what is salient in each country and its wider region. 'The tyranny of silence' described in Chapter 2 is characteristic of much of Africa, where abortion is emerging as a significant social and health problem, and social actors are unable for the most part to press governments reluctant to take action. In Mexico the question of abortion has appeared intermittently on the decision-making agenda. As elsewhere in Central and Latin America, the reality of abortion has been masked over, perpetuating existing problems. Chapter 3 explains how concerned parties are 'negotiating a hidden reality' in order to seek alternative ways out of this situation. 'Peering into Pandora's Box', Chapter 4 shows how and why conflict over abortion at times upstaged the whole process of systemic transformation as political theatre in Poland and East Central Europe. The issue of abortion, all too often divorced from a wider consideration of adequate birth control options, continues to be used as a political football by both church and state in Poland, with significant implications for women and society. Finally, Chapter 5 reviews the main findings and examines a number of major themes which weave through the study. It provides a more focused comparison between the three countries and their regions, set within a broader international context. The chapter aims at enabling the reader to understand better 'the global nature of the abortion debate', its realities and prospects, especially as it relates to public policy.

This book is intended to fill a gap in the otherwise extensive literature on abortion. It examines the emergence and construction of the abortion debate beyond the Western liberal democracies and how the Catholic Church, the most visible transnational actor in this dispute, engages this issue worldwide. Existing studies are almost entirely focused on North America and Europe, and unsuspecting readers could easily project the forces at work in those societies onto social realities in other parts of the world. Furthermore, this work gives a detailed assessment of the situation in three countries from different regions of the world and brings out the external linkages that are expanding and intensifying conflict over abortion. In addition to studying the influence of organized religion, the discourses and roles of competing actors in this dispute are analysed, along with the conditions under which abortion policies become more open to change. It is my hope that this book may appeal to scholars, those with a stake in these issues and the interested public alike, and that it may stimulate further work in this area.

The idea of this study germinated for a long time and, like many first books, had an earlier incarnation as a doctoral dissertation. I am grateful to my co-supervisors, Jason Finkle and Alison McIntosh, at the University of Michigan for their guidance and support, and to my other committee members, Yuzuru Takeshita and Kim Lane Scheppele, for their helpful comments and advice.

I have benefited immensely from having had three more years to reflect on this topic. I owe a special debt to many people I met during the course of this research with whom I had the opportunity to share information and thoughts. There are many aspects to abortion and a number of perspectives bearing on it, as recognized by the religious figure, the physician, and the women mentioned at the outset of the preface. The comparative inquiry here links up the ideas and methods of several fields to develop an informed and engaging analysis of a subject that meshes health, demography, sex, religion and politics.

I wish to express my sincere appreciation to Henryk Skolimowski for challenging me to think deeper. Also, I extend my thanks to John Slyce and Jesús Ramirez for commenting on earlier drafts of my work on Poland and Mexico, and to Prem Saxena for his useful suggestions at the end. I am grateful to Octavio Mojarro for our many conversations, and to Leopoldo Núñez and Carlos Aramburu who also helped my work proceed more smoothly in Mexico. Thanks also to Jerzy Holzer and Janina Jóźwiak for the assistance they have shown since I first started to conduct research in Poland.

I would like to acknowledge financial assistance from several sources, including the Mellon Foundation, which helped make it all possible; the Horace H. Rackham School of Graduate Studies of the University of Michigan; and the American University of Beirut for a faculty development grant that helped me finalize the manuscript. I am also grateful to Pathfinder International for providing me with office facilities in Kenya and Mexico. An earlier version of Chapter 4 appeared as an article ('Abortion Policy in Post-communist Europe: The Conflict in Poland') in the journal *Population and Development Review* (September 1995); permission to reprint parts of it has been obtained from the Population Council.

My deep appreciation and special thanks go to my brother, Ryszard, for his advice and thoughtful comments at various stages, and to my parents for their constant encouragement and for simplifying my work in Poland. My heartfelt thanks go to my wife, Lucía, for her valuable insights and tolerance, and for her enduring and loving support.

ANDRZEJ KULCZYCKI

1 A Global Policy Conundrum

INTRODUCTION

Abortion is at once a widely practised method of fertility control and a sensitive, complex and contentious issue which defies simple resolution.[1] It has sparked major controversy in the Western liberal democracies and remains a politically explosive social problem in the United States of America (USA). A review of abortion policy was initiated in former communist societies once the Soviet bloc began to disintegrate in 1989. Less noticed than these developments, abortion is an increasingly contested policy issue in a number of developing countries. This study aims in part to compare and contrast – and in effect to link – the abortion controversy globally by focusing on Kenya, Mexico and Poland, where the author has carried out extensive fieldwork.[2]

Throughout the world the issue of abortion has been considered and variously defined by government officials, political parties and administrators; ethicists and philosophers; theologians, lawyers and physicians; the family planning community, women's groups and others. Recent years have witnessed a number of changes in abortion laws, developments in medical technology, greater awareness of the widespread incidence of abortion and possible sequelae if performed unsafely, and increasing politicization of the abortion issue in many countries. These trends are likely to continue, particularly where the political environment is becoming more open and the major players in the abortion struggle are becoming more active.

Such countries include Poland and Mexico, in both of which the Roman Catholic Church, the most visible transnational actor in the abortion dispute, is opposing abortion more stridently than before. Consequently, it is desirable to examine how the Catholic Church is attempting to influence and shape abortion policy, an essentially political question with moral overtones. In other countries with sizeable and influential Catholic populations and, typically, high fertility, abortion has not yet emerged on the public agenda, but

1

there are a number of reasons for thinking that it is likely to become a hotly contested issue soon.

A good example of such a country is Kenya. During the late 1970s Kenya had the world's highest recorded birth rate; by the end of the 1980s, this had started to fall sharply and a large increase in unwanted pregnancy had been reported. The country has long been regarded as a development model for a huge continent and, despite its deteriorating political and economic situation, continues to serve as a hub for international agencies investing in the region. Kenya also has proportionately one of the largest Christian and Catholic populations in sub-Saharan Africa. Its national churches exercise a level of influence in excess of the numbers of their followers and, as in communist Poland, have been one of the few institutions to maintain a credible independent voice within a restricted civil society. The Catholic Church has spoken out against teenage pregnancy, polygamy and abortion. By the end of the 1980s a number of Kenyan family planning and medical researchers had begun to study adolescent sexuality and fertility, increasingly defined as problems and held to be responsible for a high number of abortions.

The abortion debate is particularly intense in the USA, where religion (both Catholicism and Protestant evangelism) makes its mark on society and politics most notably in the sharp schism over abortion.[3] Although historically thought of as a deeply conservative force in many world regions, those who are familiar with the Catholic Church know that for over a hundred years, successive popes have been elaborating a body of social thought on modern economic and social problems. [4] This teaching calls for greater social justice and is distinct from both liberalism and socialism.[5] Since the mid-1960s Catholicism has increasingly advocated social change. Under Pope John Paul II, the Catholic Church has championed a human rights campaign which it has explicitly linked to the ongoing quest for democratic freedoms around the world.[6] It has given institutional support to a change of regime in several countries such as Poland, the Philippines, Chile and South Korea, and exhorted leaders in Kenya, Mexico and elsewhere to initiate reform. This study underscores that the Church has extended the cause of human rights to the rights of the 'unborn'. Even if secular trends in many parts of the world have made Catholics less likely to listen to their Church hierarchy on matters pertaining to sexuality, divorce and the practices of contraception and abortion, the Catholic

Church continues to exert influence on many governments, as in Poland and, to a lesser extent, in Mexico and Kenya.

These developments have led to heightened political opposition to abortion in many countries. For example, the 1989–90 revolutions in Soviet-controlled Eastern Europe removed authoritarian regimes, opened up the prospect of resurrecting civil society, and permitted debate on many issues, including abortion. Poland's liberal abortion law quickly fell under attack from the Catholic Church, Church-backed groups and conservative politicians. This led to conflict with left-wing politicians, liberals, women's and civil libertarian groups. In Western countries, these groups typically insist on a woman's right to control her own body. In the economically developing countries, where there is much maternal morbidity and mortality associated with unsafe abortion, the concerns of such groups are both less vocalized and more basic, centring on whether women have to continue to risk their health, if not their lives, in order to regulate their own fertility.

High abortion rates are characteristic of Poland, Mexico and Kenya, the wider regions of Eastern Europe, Latin America and, increasingly, other parts of sub-Saharan Africa. They reflect the unmet need for family planning and the common recourse to abortion in the absence of contraception or in the event of contraceptive failure. In some countries, abortion is one of the most important means of birth control. This has been the case in much of East Asia and the former Soviet bloc where, as shall be discussed, government policies changed several times in response to perceptions of demographic trends, ideological preferences and political exigencies. In fact, high levels of unwanted pregnancy and unsafe abortion demand further attention and research even in Western countries, as emphasized by the World Health Organization (WHO), the United Nations Population Fund (UNFPA), and the International Planned Parenthood Federation (IPPF) in the 1990 Tbilisi Declaration.[7] These trends notwithstanding, research on abortion remains weak in developing countries and in those countries formerly in the Soviet orbit.

This book aims to help fill this gap. Abortion is figuring more prominently on the public agenda of a growing number of countries, a situation that demands careful research if attempts at resolving conflict over the issue are to be more effective than they have been so far. Comparative study of abortion is also useful precisely because abortion is a multi-dimensional contemporary issue bearing on so many other concerns, including demography, family planning, politics, law, science, ethics and religion; and because the recent growth of communications and interdependence of relations in the world means that influences are more readily transferred across countries. Consequently, how one country manages abortion can affect another country's attempts to deal with the issue. For example, the legalization of abortion in Great Britain in 1967 had repercussions elsewhere, not least in a number of Commonwealth countries because British law is the basis of their legal jurisdictions.[8] The 1973 US Supreme Court decision, *Roe* v. *Wade*, established a constitutional right to abortion before the point of viability and influenced the attempts of various countries to resolve their own abortion disputes.[9] The abortion-inducing pill RU 486 (mifepristone) marks a new method of early pregnancy termination that may alter the abortion debate in still unknown ways. It offers a non-invasive alternative to surgical abortion and works by blocking progesterone, a hormone needed to maintain pregnancy. As of late 1997, however, only Britain and Sweden had licensed mifepristone for clinical use after France had first legalized its distribution in 1988. Copies of the pill are also being used in China which is not party to international patent conventions.

This comparative analysis explores demographic and public health aspects of abortion within the wider context of the social regulation of fertility; the extent to which the awareness, interpretation and evaluation of these facts shapes abortion dynamics and laws; and the interplay of political, religious and other factors with abortion policy and practice, including the status of abortion on the political agenda and in the policymaking process. It examines the roles played by key actors engaged in the abortion debate, and particularly that of the Catholic Church as it affects abortion policy. There is a pressing need to examine these concerns, not least because of heightened activism over abortion in many parts of the world.

THE STATUS OF ABORTION RESEARCH

There is a voluminous literature on abortion, a topic that has been discussed from a variety of perspectives. For example, demographers have sought to document the incidence of abortion in various populations and the characteristics of women seeking abortions, as well as the impact of abortion on fertility rates;[10] sociologists have explored the world views of activists engaged in the abortion dispute, and the opinions of the public captured by survey data;[11] religious scholars have considered the historical treatment of abortion by the major religious teachings;[12] legal scholars have looked at the ways in which different jurisdictions have devised laws on abortion and sought to answer which approach is likely to be least contentious;[13] and some very informative general works have been written that survey the social, legal, historical, medical, ethical and cultural aspects of the issue.[14] However, writings on abortion have usually been much more partisan, invariably clouded by moral overtones, decidedly less scholarly, lacking in statistical and historical perspective, and forgetful of the multifaceted nature of the abortion issue. Also, most studies have concentrated on the ethical aspects to the controversy surrounding abortion that are not the subject of this analysis.

Despite the huge literature available on abortion and the probability that abortion has been taking place for all of human history,[15] there is a great deal that we still do not know about the empirical aspects of abortion. For example, there have been many studies assessing its incidence for which the most oft-cited global estimate is given as between 45 and 50 million abortions annually (Table 1.1). In other words, we are still far from clear about the magnitude of the phenomenon we seek to study, as well as many of its characteristics and underlying determinants, even though about one in four of all known pregnancies end in an induced abortion.

Moreover, it is not fully clear which type of policy has the greatest influence in reducing the incidence of abortion. Although this desirable goal can be realized to a considerable degree through high levels of effective contraceptive use, the abortion rate depends on other variables as well and the precise relationship between the use of abortion and contraceptive services remains unclear. In fact, the decision to end an unwanted pregnancy is usually a private matter influenced by many factors in ways still inadequately understood and affected only to a limited extent by public policies. Equally, our knowledge about the physical, emotional and mental effects of abortion on women is incomplete. Nevertheless, it is clear that first trimester abortions performed professionally under medically safe conditions carry less physical risk than bringing a pregnancy to term, and almost no risk for future fertility and pregnancy. The physical costs of an abortion may increase with the duration of pregnancy, but a review of the scientific evidence by the US Public Health Service found that existing studies 'do not provide conclusive data

Table 1.1   Global indicators of induced abortion, c. 1990

Annual number	45–50 million
Total legal	25–28 million
Total illegal	20–22 million
Abortion rate (women aged 15–44)	32–46/1,000 women
Lifetime abortion incidence (total abortion rate)	1.0–1.3/woman
Proportion of known pregnancies intentionally terminated	1 in 4 (21–28%)

Sources: S.K. Henshaw and E. Morrow, *Induced Abortion: A World Review, 1990 Supplement* (New York: Alan Guttmacher Institute, 1990); UN, *World Population Monitoring 1996: Selected Aspects of Reproductive Rights and Reproductive Health* (New York: United Nations, 1998); and WHO, *Abortion: A Tabulation of Available Data on the Frequency and Mortality of Unsafe Abortion* (Geneva: World Health Organization, 1994).

about the [mental] health effects of abortion on women'.[16] Indeed, there appears to be more evidence of relief following an abortion than of psychiatric problems, which are probably greater among women who have been denied abortion and whose 'unwanted' children may be at a developmental disadvantage.[17]

These examples point to a requirement for better informed research on abortion. The subject matter is important because of the human dimensions involved and because abortion can so often be a major contested area of public policy. Comparative study of how different societies and groups within those polities deal with abortion may highlight similarities or dissimilarities between them. It may thereby point to new insights about how various societies consider and treat abortion in the private and public domain. Below, I address five key contextual themes to illuminate the subsequent presentations and help frame the discussion. These include the demography of abortion and its interrelation with family planning and public health; the determinants of access to abortion services; the policymaking process as it pertains to abortion; the role played by the Catholic Church in the treatment of the abortion issue; and the rise of the abortion debate and its diffusion in the global arena.

FRAMEWORKS AND PERSPECTIVES

The medical demography of abortion

Contraception is usually advocated as a remedy for abortion because good quality family planning services can greatly reduce abortion rates. However, abortion itself can be no more eliminated than the controversy surrounding it can be silenced. Moreover, the relationship between abortion and contraception is complex and still inadequately documented. The demand for induced abortion within a population depends on changes in its age structure; in the proportions of women who are sexually active; in contraceptive use and efficacy; in attitudes towards unwanted pregnancy and towards single parenting; and in access to abortion services.

The most important consideration is the stage of the transfer from natural to controlled fertility of the society.[18] All countries are thought to pass through a phase of increased recourse to abortion during their demographic transition, the shift from high to low fertility (and to low mortality). The proportion of unwanted births shows an inverted U-shaped pattern and rises during the early stages of transition when there is limited ability to control fertility. It recedes as couples become more able to achieve their reproductive preferences through increased use and effectiveness of contraception. This suggests that the incidence of induced abortion is highest in countries that are in mid-transition to low fertility – those with total fertility rates (TFRs) between about 4.0 and 6.0 children per woman – and high rates of effective contraceptive use.[19] Many Latin American countries such as Mexico had such intermediate levels of fertility in the 1970s and 1980s; some African countries, such as Kenya, were entering a similar stage by the early 1990s.

Induced abortion remains the primary method of birth control in many areas of East Central Europe and the former Soviet Union that have still to move from abortion to pregnancy prevention through contraception.[20] In Latin America, birth rates have declined but high abortion rates preceded the introduction of modern contraception and continue to this day, despite very restrictive abortion laws.[21] For Mexico and Poland, improved family planning services could accelerate the shift from abortion to contraception. However, Poland has the weakest family planning infrastructure of all three countries examined here in depth. The formerly state-supported family planning agency has been unable significantly to influence reproductive behaviour, and there remains an urgent need for information, education and communication activities that could improve contraceptive efficacy. The incidence of abortion has recently increased in Kenya, as elsewhere in sub-Saharan Africa.[22] We may hypothesize that abortion rates will be small in Kenya relative to other societies that have undergone demographic transition if gains in contraceptive use precede increased resort to abortion.

Induced abortion itself is an inefficient method of fertility regulation. On average, each incidence of induced abortion averts about 0.4 births when it is not accompanied by follow-up contraceptive use, and about 0.8 births given moderately effective contraception.[23] A woman becomes fecund again sooner after an abortion than if her pregnancy had ended in a live birth. Also, some pregnancies deliberately terminated would have been aborted spontaneously.[24] For a given population, the abortion rate refers to the annual number of induced abortions expressed per 1,000 women of childbearing age. The abortion ratio is the annual number of induced abortions relative to 1,000 live births. The total abortion rate refers to the number of induced abortions which would be experienced by 1,000 women during their reproductive lifetimes, given present age-specific abortion rates.

Abortion rates are known to vary from a low of 5 abortions per 1,000 women aged 15–44 in the Netherlands, to as high as 186 abortions per 1,000 women aged 15–44 in the central region of Russia – equivalent to a lifetime average of over four abortions per woman – though this high rate has fallen since.[25] Not coincidentally, modern contraceptive use is high across all population groups in the Netherlands, where 10 per cent of known pregnancies end in abortion, and low in the former Soviet republics where most pregnancies are deliberately terminated. After peaking in the early 1980s, the US abortion rate fell a decade later to 26 per 1,000 women with 28 per cent of pregnancies ending in abortion,[26] levels still almost double those of England and Wales and higher than anywhere in Western Europe. In this region, as in North America, Australia and New Zealand, abortion rates are generally high among unmarried young women delaying childbearing, underscoring the need for improved contraceptive use. To date, young women have been more likely to marry and bring their first pregnancies to term in Central and Eastern European countries. There, overall abortion rates are higher because abortions are often obtained by older, married women who want to space or end childbirth, but who use less efficient, traditional contraceptive methods. In Japan, most abortions likewise occur among women in the older reproductive age-groups due to the low reliance on sterilization, the unavailability of birth control pills, and the financial stake physicians hold in maintaining the status quo.[27] We know very little, however, about the demography of abortion in countries where abortion is illegal. Studies tend to be limited to descriptive accounts of those women treated in hospitals for abortion-related complications.

Unsafe abortions are defined by WHO as unwanted pregnancies terminated by persons lacking the necessary skills and/or in an environment lacking the minimum medical standards.[28] Complications arising from such procedures have been and continue to be among the most neglected health and social problems. The WHO estimates about 585,000 maternal deaths occurred annually in the early 1990s, 99 per cent of them in developing countries.[29] At least 20 per cent of these deaths could be averted by access to safe abortion services and another one-third through better access to effective contraception. The global estimate is about 85,000 (or almost 20 per cent) more pregnancy-related deaths than previously believed, with estimates of abortion-related mortality halved to about 75,000 deaths per year (Table 1.2). However, this number has a large margin of error and could be as low as 50,000 or as high as 100,000. In many African countries, up to half of all maternal deaths stem from unsafe abortion, but the absolute number of such deaths is thought to be greater in South Asia. For each death, many more women suffer injuries and complications that may lead to permanent, long-term disabilities. The treatment of incomplete and septic abortions imposes a major burden on scarce hospital resources in many poor countries. Knowledge of such health sequelae of unsafe abortion is pertinent to informed debate on this topic and may even transform policy. This is why, for example, a number of Kenyan researchers and gynaecologists have sought to publicize the widespread incidence of illegal abortion and its public health costs.

The safety of the abortion procedure depends primarily on the choice of method used, the conditions under which it is performed, the skill of the abortion provider, and certain characteristics of the woman herself such as her general health, age, parity and stage of pregnancy. Whereas, for developing countries, WHO estimates the risk of death at 1 in 250 abortion procedures, in developed countries

Table 1.2   Global and regional estimates of clandestine and unsafe abortions and associated mortality

Region	Number of clandestine abortions (millions)	Clandestine abortions per 1,000 women of 15–49 years	Deaths from unsafe abortions	Case fatality per 100 clandestine abortions	Risk of death from clandestine abortions	Deaths from clandestine abortions per 100,000 live births
World	20	15	70 000	0.4	1 in 300	49
Less developed regions	17.6	17	69 000	0.4	1 in 250	55
More developed regions*	2.3	8	600	0.03	1 in 3 700	4
Africa	3.7	26	23 000	0.6	1 in 150	83
Asia*	9.2	12	40 000	0.4	1 in 250	47
Latin America and Caribbean	4.6	41	6 000	0.1	1 in 800	48

Figures may not add to totals because of rounding.

* Japan is included in the total for the more developed regions, but is excluded from the regional estimate for Asia.

Source: Adapted from WHO, *Abortion: A Tabulation of Available Data on the Frequency and Mortality of Unsafe Abortion* (Geneva: World Health Organization, 1994).

Note: The World Health Organization's tabulations consider all abortions that are not legally sanctioned to be unsafe. However, such abortions may be carried out by physicians who are more likely to use less hazardous techniques than in the past, so that the terms are not necessarily synonymous. Accordingly, this table distinguishes between clandestine and unsafe abortions where appropriate.

it has declined to as low as 0.4 cases per 100,000 procedures, less than that from an injection of penicillin. In the US, for example, the case-fatality rate fell by about 90 per cent between 1972 and 1987, making complications related to the anaesthesia used the most common cause of abortion-related deaths. The risk of death from childbirth is at least 11 times higher, and 30 times higher than for abortions up to eight weeks of gestation. Mortality risks from abortions performed at 16–20 weeks or over are substantially higher than the risk associated with procedures carried out at 8 weeks or less (Table 1.3).

Abortion in the early stages of pregnancy has become safer in many countries with the introduction of vacuum aspiration, otherwise known as suction curettage. This relies on a vacuum to dis-

Table 1.3   Legal abortion and mortality: Death rates and relative risks
by selected characteristics, United States of America, 1972–87

Characteristic	Mortality rate per 100,000 procedures	Relative risk and 95% confidence interval
Age (years)		
15–19	1.0	1.0 Referent
20–24	1.3	1.3 (0.9, 1.8)
25–44	1.6	1.5 (1.1, 2.1)
Gestational Age (weeks)		
up to 8	0.4	1.0 Referent
9–10	0.8	2.1 (1.3, 3.3)
11–12	1.4	3.7 (2.3, 5.8)
13–15	2.9	7.7 (5.0, 11.7)
16–20	9.3	24.5 (18.6, 32.3)
21+	12.0	31.5 (22.2, 44.5)
Type of procedure		
Suction and sharp curettage	0.5	1.0 Referent
Dilatation and evacuation	3.7	6.8 (4.9, 9.5)
Instillation	7.1	13.0 (9.7, 17.5)
Hysterectomy-hysterotomy	51.6	95.0 (69.6, 129.5)

The relative risk refers to the association between the specified characteristic
and abortion. It is expressed as a ratio given here in relation to a value of
one for the lowest risk for that group of characteristics. The confidence
interval contains the relative risk of interest within a 95 per cent degree
of confidence. The upper and lower bounds of this interval are listed in
parentheses.

Source: H.W. Lawson, A. Frye, H.K. Atrash, J.C. Smith, H.B. Shulman
and M. Ramick, 'Abortion mortality, United States, 1972 through 1987',
American Journal of Obstetrics and Gynecology, 171 (1994), 5, 1365–72.

lodge the embryo through a cannula. With manual vacuum aspiration (MVA), the vacuum is generated by a hand-held syringe rather
than an electric pump. Vacuum aspiration is among the safest of
surgical procedures in rich countries. It is a simpler and more cost-
effective method than dilatation and curettage (D&C, also known
as sharp curettage), particularly for treating incomplete abortion.[30]
This condition is often associated with infections and requires evacuation of the embryo, uterine lining, and the placenta. However, in
most poor countries it is still treated by D&C, which involves di-
lating the cervix to allow insertion of surgical instruments used to
remove the contents of the uterus.

Although traumatic damage to the uterus can affect future fertility, suction curettage abortion does not increase the chance of secondary infertility. Also, an uncomplicated termination of pregnancy does not have any adverse outcomes on later reproduction or on the risk of breast cancer.[31] For abortions performed between 13 and 20 weeks, dilatation and evacuation (D&E) is commonly used and involves greater dilatation of the cervix than does a conventional vacuum aspiration. It is also safer than intrauterine instillation of saline, prostaglandin or urea, the previous method of choice. Hysterotomies and hysterectomies, once widely used for late-term abortions, are associated with the highest mortality risks (Table 1.3) and have been discredited for such purpose.

The antiprogestin mifepristone (RU 486) can make early abortion more private and convenient for women by offering a medical, non-surgical procedure. It may be used through the ninth week of pregnancy and is most effective when taken with a prostaglandin such as misoprostol that causes strong uterine contractions. Mifepristone may also treat a variety of disorders and serve as an efficacious emergency (post-coital) contraceptive because it can hinder conception.[32] However, its abortifacient role makes it one of the most controversial medications of recent times and there remain major political obstacles to its acceptance. Another effective and cheaper way of medically terminating an early pregnancy involves the combination of two medicines readily available at low cost in many parts of the world. In this two-step procedure, pregnancy is interrupted by methotrexate, better known as a cancer treatment interfering with cell growth and division. To expel the foetus, clients return several days later to be given misoprostol, also used in the mifepristone procedure and otherwise as an ulcer medicine.[33] Medical methods of termination take longer to act than surgical procedures and require medical supervision in case of method failure or continued bleeding.

Access to abortion services

The legal status of abortion is a key determinant of access to abortion services, particularly their safety. This has often been differentiated according to the developmental stages of foetal life, national and local legal systems, as well as between different branches of the law (criminal, constitutional, family, civil and common law). The latest available estimates (from the early 1990s) suggest that

38 per cent of the world's population live in countries where early abortion is legally available on request of the pregnant woman.[34] In total, about 63 per cent of the world's population live under laws that (theoretically) permit access to abortion on request or on a wide variety of grounds. It is also noteworthy that where abortion is legal in most circumstances, there is no consensus as to how late an abortion may legally be performed. Figure 1.1 presents a detailed summary of laws governing the permissibility of induced abortion, broken down into the percentages of countries and of people affected worldwide.

An examination of abortion statutes and penal codes alone would suggest that one-quarter (25 per cent) of the world's population live in countries where abortion is illegal under any circumstances, or authorized only to save the life of a pregnant woman. Where abortion is banned, however, it is still usually legal under general principles of common law, as in Egypt; due to the prevailing legal interpretation, as in Colombia and Indonesia; or due to certain allowances under codes of medical ethics, public health or social welfare.[35] Such exceptions reveal that about 4 per cent of the world's population live in countries that do not permit a pregnancy to be terminated if it endangers the life of a woman. Implicit provisions sometimes allow abortion in the event of all so-called 'hard cases', where pregnancy stems from a criminal act, may result in genetic defects, or seriously endangers a woman's health. Nevertheless, where abortion is illegal, it is typically carried out in unhygienic conditions that cause high rates of morbidity and death.

A worldwide trend towards the liberalization of abortion laws began in the 1950s as most Eastern European countries followed the lead of the Soviet Union, predating such changes in Western Europe (outside of Scandinavia) and North America by at least a decade.[36] During the 1960s and 1970s, abortion reached the political agenda of most of the Western liberal democracies, where it was legalized last in predominantly Catholic countries. Ireland and Malta alone retain strong restrictions, prompting many women to travel abroad to obtain an abortion, a phenomenon often referred to as 'abortion tourism'. In Asia abortion was legalized on broad grounds primarily out of demographic concern by India (1971) and China (1957), as done even earlier by the USSR (1955) and Japan (1948).[37] Several Asian Muslim states, notably Bangladesh, Indonesia and Malaysia, now permit menstrual regulation (the evacuation of the uterine contents by suction, just after a missed

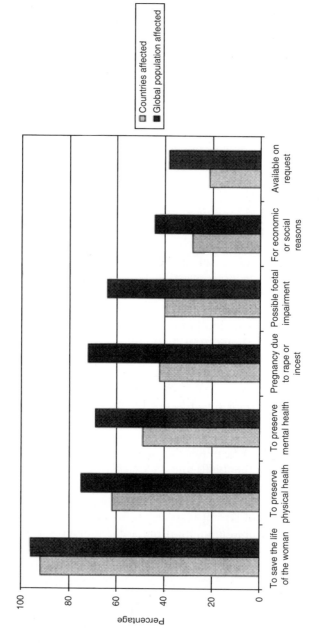

Figure 1.1 Legal grounds for abortion worldwide

menstrual period)[38] and distinguish it from abortion, which remains legally restricted except to save the life of the pregnant woman. By contrast, nearly all Latin American, African and Middle Eastern countries maintain highly restrictive laws on abortion dating back to colonial times.

Despite the common focus on the law by nearly all analysts, the actual implementation of abortion laws and the degree to which they are enforced is more central in determining the availability and use of abortion services than the law *per se*. For example, Mexico may be characterized as a 'lapsed law' country where abortion is nominally illegal but services are often readily available, seemingly with the acquiescence of the government, and there are few prosecutions. The quality of the abortions women obtain varies widely; although relatively safe, even though not always affordable, abortion services are available in all major Latin American cities.[39] Indeed, laws and policies may have a greater impact on the safety of abortion services than on either the actual process of obtaining an abortion itself or on the resultant incidence of abortion. In Romania, for example, a six-fold increase in abortion mortality ensued after abortion and the importation of contraceptives were prohibited in 1966 to encourage population growth.[40] Throughout the 1980s, abortion-related deaths accounted for at least 84 per cent of all maternal deaths, and in 1984 the WHO reported 449 such deaths, six times the number of maternal deaths from all other causes, which had declined over the same period. Many more women were permanently injured, with official government statistics indicating a higher abortion rate than in any Western European country where abortion was legal.

In many settings, low socio-economic status is a stronger barrier to abortion than is the legal status. The rich and socially advantaged can invariably obtain safe abortions, for which they may travel abroad. Also, legislative reforms in many countries may not be matched by an adequate service delivery due to such reasons as the refusal of physicians to perform abortions, bureaucratic requirements, and a lack of trained providers or of affordable services, particularly in rural areas. This creates inequalities of access to legal abortion in rich countries such as the USA and Austria, as well as in poorer countries such as India and Zambia where relatively few people are aware of the legality of the procedure. In the USA in 1992, 84 per cent of all counties and 94 per cent of non-metropolitan counties had no abortion provider, with 18 per cent fewer hospitals offering such services than in 1988.[41] Clearly, access to safe abortion services may be affected by social attitudes beyond those of service providers, as well as by authorization procedures, administrative circumstances, a lack of appropriate technology, and poor transport and referral networks.

The abortion policymaking process

There is an enormous amount of opinion poll data on abortion in the liberal democracies. Community attitudes towards abortion provide some direction in policymaking and, to a limited extent, in making moral judgments, but such surveys are notoriously sensitive to the wording of questions and to the researcher's values. Opinions about abortion are frequently marked by ambivalence and a gap between stated beliefs and actual practice. In any case, public attitudes are of little significance to policymaking in societies where political participation is restricted. This is one reason for focusing on the proximate decision-makers and elites influential in the abortion policy field.

Abortion policies have been instituted as a result of a variety of pressures such as socialist ideology, feminism and religious beliefs. The process by which abortion laws and policies have been formulated differs even more across countries. In Western democracies there has generally been a long and complex debate involving legislatures, political parties, administrative bureaucracies, judiciaries, as well as interest groups.[42] In the USA, Canada and the former West Germany, judicial decisions have been the determining factor and the focus of subsequent challenges; in England, France and elsewhere, parliament has been the main forum; and decisions by referendums have played central roles in Italy and Ireland. Italian citizens voted in 1981 to keep a more liberal law passed three years earlier. In Ireland, where Catholicism remains strong and conservative, voters rejected liberalizing existing restrictions in 1983 when they elevated the right to life of the 'unborn' to a level equal to that of the prospective mother. In 1992 they again rejected a proposal to extend the grounds for abortion, but approved of making it legal to travel abroad for an abortion and to receive information about the procedure.[43]

Across countries, we consistently find similar actors engaged in the abortion debate, albeit with different levels of influence and some variation in their agendas and strategies. They include the state, the medical profession, religious organizations (most notably the Catholic Church), women's groups and, increasingly, family planning agencies. Such groups may resort to a variety of strategies so as to influence abortion policy. They may, for example, use data to show the scale of unsafe abortion and the costs associated with it, or draw attention to policy solutions found elsewhere. However, agenda-setting demands time, effort and the mobilization of resources. The process can be greatly advanced when problems, proposed solutions and favourable political forces become joined at critical times.[44] Such 'windows' of opportunity to change policy may be generated by events that focus attention on abortion. For example, debate was accelerated in the USA and in several European countries by 'the thalidomide tragedy' in the early 1960s, when a new medication prescribed to pregnant women caused severe birth defects. An epidemic of rubella (German measles) promptly refocused public attention on the abortion issue because of the increased likelihood of foetal deformities if rubella is contracted during pregnancy.[45] These widely reported episodes occurred during a time of growing re-evaluation of the quality of life, and played a major role in transforming public and medical opinion about abortion.

This illustrates how new perspectives can bring attention to particular problems. When a situation becomes widely perceived as unsatisfactory and needing action, conflicting opinions are invariably presented as to how it should be remedied. The issue may be considered in the policy process, and policy choices may be proposed and debated. However, much of the American and European literature on agenda-building focuses on legislatures which are less important in many economically developing countries where issues are neither so widely debated, nor contested. The ruling elites are in a dominant position to shape policy precisely because they hold key power positions, play a central role in addressing (or abstaining from addressing) abortion as well as other troublesome aspects of social life, and help bridge outside values with traditional ones. The elites bring their perceptions, commitments and resources to bear on the abortion issue. They may argue for a particular policy alternative, or for its postponement or suppression. They may also seek consensus among those policy options proposed by various groups.

Kenyans in recent years have suffered the erosion of civil liberties, but Catholic and other churchmen have not refrained from criticizing the government's drift towards one-party rule and sub-jugation of legal authority. The government, not wanting to risk greater societal alienation, cannot idly ignore the pronouncements of religious groups on abortion and matters pertaining to sexuality. Nonetheless, in places such as Kenya, we may be witnessing the beginning of an abortion reform movement as a number of concerned physicians have started to address the abortion issue. They are try-ing to place abortion on the agenda by focusing attention (where it has not been before) on the health costs associated with treating the consequences of unsafe and illegally procured abortions. Locating abortion in medical discourse may also empower physicians to the detriment of women and not only restrict the power of other social actors, notably husbands and religious groups, or state institutions.

The abortion policy process is ongoing and is far from settled in many states. Controversy may continue long after policies are de-bated and laws are enacted. Attitudes and policies may be influ-enced by the divergent values and perceptions different groups bring to the abortion dispute, and by changes in organizational and in-stitutional arrangements, such as the position of women in society and the role of gender-power relations in the formation of public policy. As emerges from this study, however, the Catholic Church, feminists and politicians alike tend to concentrate their resources in this debate on modifying abortion laws.

The abortion debate is enmeshed in conflict that involves tradi-tional political tactics such as lobbying legislators and mobilizing publics. It also involves a struggle over meaning and, specifically, over what should be the goals of abortion policy. The players in this debate are passionately arguing not just over abortion *per se*; their disagreements reflect very different understandings of the foetus, of the woman, and indeed of how the world should be structured. Hence the conduct of the abortion debate is greatly complicated by the use of a number of competing discourses. These include the differ-ent languages adopted by the Catholic Church, by less well known opponents of abortion, by women's rights groups, civil rights groups and medical circles. To take but two examples, the 1980s witnessed the emergence of two relatively new vocabularies in the abortion debate and the attempt to integrate each into legal theory and praxis. One centred on the concept of 'reproductive rights', a broad pol-itical demand for full female reproductive and sexual autonomy; the other focused on the 'unborn child', taken one step further in Poland with the discursive construction of the 'conceived child'. In the mid-1990s, US activists also applied the term 'partial-birth abortion' to a rarely used late-term procedure. The use of such rhetorical strategies may transform the way abortion is thought of and defined.

Since the late 1980s, Kenya, Mexico and Poland have been characterized by turbulent political environments. The ability of interest groups to exploit this situation increases their chances of ensuring that the issue of abortion obtains access to the governmental agenda where it will be more seriously addressed by decision-makers. Systemic changes offer new opportunities and challenges for organized groups to redefine the way abortion is considered. For example, abortion figured on the political agenda of most Central and Eastern European societies following the overthrow of authoritarian regimes in 1989. By far the most bitter controversy took place in Poland where Catholic bishops and right-wing politicians, encouraged by Pope John Paul II, moved swiftly to outlaw abortion. This had become an accepted medical procedure among many Polish women and physicians after the state had sanctioned its practice in 1956.

The Catholic Church and abortion

Beyond its central religious role, the Catholic Church may be considered a pressure group with a well-organized constituency among its most devoted followers.[46] Like any large institution, it may attempt to influence governmental decisions that concern its juridical or economic status. Of greater significance to this investigation, the Church's mission demands that it should speak out on moral and social issues, such as abortion. The Catholic Church remains the most highly organized religious group and one of the most influential social institutions in the world. It is a hierarchical organization with an extensive supranational network, able to exert influence on a number of social and political issues defined as having a moral nature.[47] Within each country, a bishop typically serves as the head of a commission concerned with all matters pertaining to family life, a rubric under which pastoral concern for abortion is often considered. The commission's work is reviewed by the national episcopal conference, a body which may serve as a lobbying group for influencing public policy. These bishops' conferences became widespread after the Second Vatican Council (Vatican II, 1962–65) facilitated greater collegiality within the Church.[48]

There is a long history to Catholic Church thinking and official teaching on abortion. While this is the product of considerable reflection on abortion, it is to a large degree inseparable from the way the Church has considered human sexuality, marriage and motherhood, and its longstanding opposition to birth control, a dogma inherited from earlier times when death rates were much greater and high fertility was essential for human survival. As with other religious institutions and like most nation-states until very recently, the pronatalism of the Church establishment has also rested in a desire to have more communicants so as to increase its own influence. In addition, abortion is taken to be at odds with Catholic teaching on family values and the 'family' institution as the core of social life. This is a constant theme of Pope John Paul II, as expressed in the Vatican's Charter of Family Rights (1983) and frequently restated during the International Year of the Family declared for 1994 by the Catholic Church as well as the United Nations (UN).[49]

All these elements enter the abortion debate, but the core of the Church's concern rests with the right to life of the foetus (the 'unborn') which is considered more important than the rights of the pregnant woman. This view is identified most closely with the *magisterium*, the teaching authority of the Church centred on the Pope and bishops, who consider it the basis for Catholic orthodoxy on the issue. However, many divergent arguments exist within the Catholic tradition, and the Church is made up of all its members, many of whom hold different views on this matter from the senior hierarchy. To take the most obvious area of contention, many Catholic theologians, scholars and churchmen, including at least some prelates, do not necessarily agree that the 'official' teaching should hold if the life of the pregnant woman is at stake. This underscores the difficulty of speaking about an exclusively Catholic position on abortion even if, in a narrow and traditional sense, the Church has been regarded as the pope and the bishops.

As is common knowledge, there is a marked gap in the rich countries between the practice of the Catholic laity and the teaching of the hierarchy over contraception. By the early 1990s, for example, US Catholics were as likely as non-Catholics to use contraception and to have low fertility, although religious groups may vary in patterns of method use.[50] Italy, where the Vatican is situated, and Catholic Spain had the lowest birth rates in Europe. The average number of children born to a woman in Brazil, the world's largest Catholic nation, fell within a generation from 5.8 in 1970 to 2.3 in 1993, and stands at below replacement level in the more developed south. Regarding abortion, those most religiously active are more likely to accept official teaching; but, as a group, Catholic women resort to abortion as often as non-Catholics.[51] Also, Catholic respondents exhibit a range of opinions on the morality and permissibility of abortion even if they tend to be more critical than their fellow citizens.

Religious teachings often serve to give helpful moral guidance, but, despite their strong influence on abortion attitudes and laws, religious traditions do not offer historically consistent positions on abortion. The world's major religions have adopted a variety of opinions on abortion. The Catholic Church has always taken a serious view of abortion, although its reasoning has changed over time along with its engagement over the issue.[52] Historically, Church doctrine did not consider abortion to be a grave sin before the foetus was infused with a soul, a moment known as ensoulment, or animation. This was taken to occur at quickening, the point at which a woman could feel movements from the foetus, typically around 16–18 weeks of gestation. This meant that the position of the Church, common law and the practices of women tended to correspond.[53]

In the nineteenth century, religious, medical and legal authorities re-examined the meaning of quickening. Pope Pius IX altered Church teaching in 1869 by removing the distinction between the 'formed' (ensouled) and 'unformed' foetus and decreeing that Catholics performing an abortion at any stage of pregnancy would be excommunicated (a punishment extended in 1917 to include the woman undergoing an abortion). Pius XI reiterated this teaching in his 1930 encyclical on Christian marriage and family life, *Casti Connubii*. Although this encyclical is better known for its denunciation of contraceptives, it also condemned therapeutic abortion on the grounds that it led to the killing of innocent life. Most recently, John Paul II has strongly and repeatedly stressed that human life is sacred and inviolable from the moment of conception, and should be respected and protected as such. His eleventh encyclical, *Evangelium Vitae* ('The Gospel of Life', released in 1995), categorically rejects abortion and depicts its legalization and acceptance in Western countries as symptomatic of an encroaching 'culture of death'.[54]

The success with which the Church opposes abortion is qualified by two major considerations. Firstly, while its doctrine is basically uniform, a more important variable determining its influence may be its strength in relation to other societal institutions. Recent years have witnessed growing activism on the part of feminist and other interest groups that have generally opposed the Church's position on birth control and abortion. Nevertheless, the Church is an old hand at politics. In the USA, for instance, it has provided vital energy, organizational assistance and direction to the 'right-to-life' movement. [55] In so doing, it has cooperated with a number of Protestant churches. Between 1917 and 1992 anti-clerical constitutional provisions prevented the Mexican Catholic Church from exercising as strong an influence in public life as in most Latin American countries. However, it commanded a level of presence and social credibility that no opposition party or group could maintain. Some of the Church's agenda is also realized by religious societies, in recent years including the elite and secretive organizations, Opus Dei and the Knights of Malta. Opus Dei (Latin for 'Work of God') promotes traditional Catholic values and fidelity to Church authority and doctrine, and is an especially controversial organization. By the early 1990s it had 75,000 members worldwide, including many influential Catholics in governmental, professional and business positions, particularly in Spain and Latin America. It also had at least 1,500 priests and remains very clerical.[56]

A second factor is the realization that, despite the common perception that the institutional church speaks with a single voice, there is a considerable variance in its engagement in the abortion dispute both within and between countries, as has been the case over contraception. In Kenya, for instance, the Catholic Church is a major actor in the struggle for a more open public sphere and accountable government. The bishops have also come into conflict with government attempts to extend family planning, although they have diluted their opposition to the provision of contraceptives *per se*. In the USA, despite the strong stand taken by Church leaders, many Catholics oppose restrictive abortion laws. This includes one small but vocal advocacy group, Catholics for a Free Choice.[57] Under the former regime in Poland, the Church acted as an umbrella for the activities of the democratic opposition. The 1978 election of a Polish Pope – the first non-Italian pope since 1523 – increased the religious fervour of his compatriots, for whom nationalism and Catholicism had become closely tied. In the immediate post-communist period, the Polish Church attempted to reassert its influence over its followers and in public life, notably through its campaign to delegalize abortion and in its opposition to contraceptives. Along with the Holy See, it sought to set a precedent for the former socialist countries, as well as Catholic Western European countries which had recently liberalized abortion, by reversing a very permissive abortion statute. The Pope and his more militant advisers also wanted to suggest a model for non-European countries considering abortion policy changes.

This determined stand reflects the arguments made by many Church leaders against Western support for family planning programmes in Africa, Latin America and Asia.[58] Their efforts have made governments of countries with a large proportion of Catholics, and particularly those whose leaders are committed Catholics, reluctant to propose population policies that promote fertility reduction, particularly attempts to legalize abortion. For example, the Church has been for centuries a powerful force in the Philippines where 85 per cent of the people are baptized Catholics. Cory Aquino, a devout Catholic who took over from the ousted Marcos regime in the 1986 People's Power revolution, was institutionally beholden to Catholic bishops for political support. She promptly pushed through constitutional provisions whereby 'the state recognizes the sanctity of family life' and is required to protect 'the life of the unborn from conception'.[59]

Changes have occurred in the structure of Christian churches in both Africa and Latin America. One can point to a definite 'inculturation' of Christianity, or the blending of its Western practices with local ideas and cultural traditions. Both continents have also witnessed an infusion of new missionary churches, some of which are fundamentalist, pentecostal or millenarian in character. They are usually strongly opposed to abortion but tend not to exert a significant influence on how this matter is considered by policymakers. The mainstream Protestant churches tolerate abortion when the health or life of the woman is threatened. However, Protestant churches in general are deeply divided about the moral dimensions of abortion. They tend to avoid taking a categorical stand on the beginning of life and often adopt an ambivalent approach to abortion. On the other hand, the Religious Coalition for Abortion Rights is an advocacy group in the USA made up of 35 religious denominations, primarily Protestant, that oppose efforts to restrict access to abortion.

Pope John Paul II has accorded high priority to the abortion issue. He is a bold and articulate pontiff who has developed a dynamic and vigorous style of papacy, much more visible than that of his predecessors. He has reimposed ecclesiastical conservatism and doctrinal orthodoxy, as reflected in the new universal catechism of the Catholic Church.[60] The historic tension between the administrative core of the Church in Rome and the principle of collegiality is evident in John Paul II's simultaneous stress on hierarchical centralism and his upgrading of the status of the national and regional conferences of bishops that confer about a wide range of issues. John Paul II has also stressed pastoral care and strongly reaffirmed the message of social justice carried in Catholic social teaching,[61] which has received less international attention than it deserves.

My interviews with senior churchmen and Catholic scholars in Poland suggest that, as Bishop Wojtyła, the future pope influenced Paul VI's encyclical *Humanae Vitae* ('Of Human Life', published in 1968). Indeed, echoes of Wojtyła's earlier pastoral and ethical treatise on human sexuality, *Love and Responsibility*,[62] can be found in that deeply controversial encyclical which condemned the use of 'artificial' contraceptives as 'intrinsically wrong'.[63] The encyclical restated that every sexual act should occur in marriage and that induced abortion, even if for therapeutic reasons, was illicit. John Paul II has long been one of the strongest defenders of *Humanae Vitae* and has sought to enshrine its teaching as unambiguous Church doctrine. He has reiterated traditional Church doctrine on all matters pertaining to reproduction and family life, making unequivocal statements on abortion in a number of documents and during many of the 80 overseas papal trips he had made by 1997.

The rise and diffusion of the abortion debate in the global arena

Before the middle of the twentieth century, abortion was rarely discussed in public, if at all. It lay at the margins of issue consideration for many reasons. These included widespread pronatalist beliefs; the inferior status of women; repressive attitudes toward sexuality, especially that of women; and knowledge that abortion procedures were then quite dangerous and caused many deaths. Any question of abortion policy reform was closely supervised by religious, medical and state institutions.

Abortion has emerged as an issue on the world stage due to a host of pressures. Foremost among these have been social changes, particularly in gender roles, as more women have entered the formal labour market and have become self-supporting; and the emergence of stronger feminist groups than hitherto that have demanded acceptance of a woman's right to legal abortion. Along with the growing emphasis on self-determination and individualism, the 'sexual revolution' in the increasingly pluralistic populations of Western Europe and North America acted as a catalyst in undermining religious teachings and social mores on sexuality, birth control and abortion. In the 1960s and 1970s these countries witnessed the organization of vocal and articulate movements promoting the legalization of abortion, a cause legitimized by strong support from medical associations. The success of these reform movements in Great Britain and the USA in particular hastened the trend in more affluent countries towards liberalization of the grounds under which abortion is legally permitted in the early stages of pregnancy. These developments provoked a strong reaction, particularly from the Catholic Church, and gave rise to anti-abortion lobbies which had some success in reversing measures that broadened the provision of abortion services, especially in the USA during the 1980s.

Abortion has also been redefined as a problem because of increased awareness of the rapid growth of world population and of the health problems linked to unsafe abortion, allied with the desire to ameliorate these conditions. The simpler and safer technologies developed to perform abortion and to treat unsafe abortion have enabled better quality services to be more widely available. This has encouraged medical professionals to consolidate another area of professional autonomy.[64] It has also broadened reproductive choices for women, greatly expanded a few years earlier by the introduction of oral contraceptives and intrauterine devices (IUDs).

In general, abortion is a subject of much greater moral, emotional and legal concern to Americans than to most Europeans. In the USA abortion has figured constantly in the headlines since it was legalized in 1973. Interest groups have moved strategically in raising awareness, mobilizing supporters and pushing for judicial, legislative and executive action regarding abortion. Intent on reversing the legalization of abortion, the US National Conference of Catholic Bishops helped establish the National Right to Life Committee, the largest 'pro-life' organization in the country, and developed the 1975 Pastoral Plan for Pro-Life Activities, which brought the Church more directly into the political arena. Soon afterwards, the 'New Right' coalition, a powerful religious and political movement made up of born-again Protestants, conservative Catholics and right-wing Republicans, successfully used the abortion issue as a grassroots organizing tool and assured critical support for Presidents Reagan and Bush throughout the 1980s.[65] Both men cultivated close ties with the Catholic Church and presided over a growing number of restrictions on abortion and family planning services. Their strong support for the anti-abortion movement encouraged an intensification of debate that coincided with a number of violent attacks by extremists on clinics providing abortion services.[66] A ban on the importation of mifepristone made its French manufacturer and its German parent delay seeking marketing approval for the pill in many countries.

The US government exercises a major impact on global considerations of abortion due to its political, economic and cultural influence, including its disproportionately significant role in supporting international family planning efforts. During the 1980s these became strongly embroiled in the controversy surrounding abortion. At the 1984 International Conference on Population held in Mexico City, the US government, the largest population aid donor in the world through its Agency for International Development (USAID),[67] declared that population growth was 'of itself, a neutral phenomenon'. This dramatic turnaround in international population policy reflected the success of the anti-abortion lobby whose agenda extended to cutting back support for family planning, both in the US and overseas. The so-called 'Mexico City policy' also strongly echoed Vatican views on family planning, abortion and global population concerns.[68] It prohibited US government funding for any multilateral or non-governmental agencies that 'perform or actively promote abortion as a method of family planning', even if they did so with funds from non-USAID sources.[69] This stifled abortion research and adversely affected the willingness of family planning and health clinics to treat women with incomplete abortions. It also provided an expedient excuse for withdrawing support from two well-established international family planning agencies: UNFPA, on the pretext that it supported a family planning programme in China which included coercive abortions, and IPPF, which continued to support national affiliates that provided abortion services, since each made its own spending decisions.[70] These policies remained in force until they were rescinded nearly a decade later.[71]

The Catholic Church is another key influence on the way abortion is considered in many countries, as elucidated in the following chapters. Pope John Paul II, a towering moral authority on the world scene, has used his office to project his categorical support for unborn life and has encouraged legislative and political initiatives to that end. Many bishops have stressed the Church's doctrinal stand over abortion and have fostered opposition to the provision of abortion services. Such a strong stance can influence the policy positions adopted by states regardless of whether lay Catholics who agree with such views hold key governmental posts.

Beyond the influences of the US government and the Catholic Church, feminist groups constitute the third critical mover in the internationalization of the abortion debate. The women's movement gathered strength at the international level during the UN Decade for Women that began and ended with conferences at Mexico City, 1975, and Nairobi, 1985, respectively.[72] A number of 'women's health' advocates have since sought to enshrine the right to reproductive choice into international law and policy, particularly in a series of important UN conferences on human rights (held in Vienna, 1993), population and development (Cairo, 1994), and the status of women (Beijing, 1995). They have had some success in influencing international family planning organizations. Whereas UNFPA officially holds no 'position' with regard to abortion beyond its stated concern over the health consequences of unsafe abortion, the IPPF committed itself more strongly and adopted a new charter implicitly endorsing a woman's right to terminate an unwanted pregnancy.[73]

The abortion debate has moved beyond its two epicentres in the USA and Rome. It now permeates many areas of the world, although it does not necessarily take the same form in different settings. It is further fuelled and sustained by the increasing interaction of cultures and belief systems. Ideas and central issues are now rapidly diffused by the global revolution in communications. The international mass media has dichotomized the issue as one between those 'in favour of' and those 'against' abortion, and images and reports of the very public and divisive US abortion controversy have been seen and discussed elsewhere.

Well-organized groups from the economically advanced nations, primarily the USA, have sought to nurture similar bodies overseas. Groups have to some extent tapped into existing networks such as those of the Catholic Church, medical organizations and family planning agencies. A number of international linkages have been developed,[74] although these remain loose-knit. Secondary waves of influence are now evident. For example, anti-abortion activists from Poland have joined up with those from the USA to work in neighbouring countries. The US-based Human Life International, founded by a Catholic priest, financed and helped organize in 1994 the first major anti-abortion conference in Russia, co-sponsored with the Russian Orthodox Church.[75] In Zambia, Human Life International has for many years been active in an attempt to reverse the first liberal abortion law passed in sub-Saharan Africa.[76] More than anywhere else on the continent, Catholic lay groups have gained enough strength to disrupt family planning activities and to foil moves to improve access to abortion services. As we shall see, the Mexican group Pro-Vida has likewise sought to strengthen a doctrinal Catholic position by fostering similar organizations elsewhere in Latin America. However, linkages between groups remain poorly developed, not least because of profound differences between them. This is the case both within and across countries, as shown in the following chapters. The ability of groups from all sides of the abortion debate to influence developments in the economically developing countries is further hindered by political, legal and cultural barriers. There are also difficulties in negotiating financial and organizational resources, including a problem in finding committed allies able to devote time to such efforts.

Several Asian states liberalized their abortion laws once they decided their family planning services were incomplete without the provision of abortion. India legalized abortion four years after Britain, but remains the only South Asian country to have done so. Abortion has played a major role in the fertility declines of Japan, China and South Korea, where strong ruling elites legalized abortion after having decided on an economic need to reduce population growth.[77] There have been only minor religious and ideological obstacles in these countries, perhaps because Hindus and Buddhists believe in rebirth which mitigates the tenet that abortion is a wrong.[78] Moreover, ecclesiastical structures and official doctrines are not as important as in Catholicism. Political participation has been restricted in these societies, pre-empting potential controversy over a permissive abortion policy. Beyond the Arabic heartland, Asian Islamic countries generally provide menstrual regulation services as a public health measure, thereby circumventing the need for any changes in the criminal code. In addition, the lack of a consensus in Islam on the status of abortion in the first four months of pregnancy has mollified opposition to such a move from more patriarchal interpretations of the religion.[79] Turkey and Tunisia began to liberalize their abortion laws in the 1960s, although access to services can be restricted in practice.

Broader legal developments are now playing a role in bringing up debate on abortion. Many states have come to accept a more pragmatic approach to criminal law and realize that restrictive abortion codes are to a large extent unenforceable and discriminatory against poor women in particular. International developments in the areas of law and the principles of human rights, such as the Convention on the Elimination of All Forms of Discrimination Against Women (adopted by the UN General Assembly in 1979), have instilled greater awareness of the gender discriminatory nature of many institutional practices. This has led to more countries adopting constitutional and human rights provisions that promote gender equality. It has also facilitated reassessment of what became known as 'reproductive rights', a rallying cry under which feminists from more affluent countries increasingly subsumed the demand for legal abortion.

The New York-based International Women's Health Coalition and the Women's Environment and Development Organization are two groups that have effectively pushed this demand, strengthened women's health groups, and built linkages with health care organizations and population agencies. Such activities have focused attention on developing policies that integrate abortion services with other areas of reproductive health including family planning, maternal and child health, and sexually transmitted diseases. The International Women's Health Coalition organized two symposiums on the theme of unwanted pregnancy and women's reproductive health immediately after the triennial meetings of the International Federation of Gynecology and Obstetrics (FIGO) in Berlin, 1985, and Rio de Janeiro, 1988.[80] At Rio, a petition signed by 2,000 FIGO members prompted the French health minister to call mifepristone 'the moral property of women' and to order its production and distribution to be resumed after French and US anti-abortion groups threatened to organize a boycott of the manufacturer's products.[81] Vocal physicians' lobbies exist to deny women access to legal and medically safe abortion in some countries, but groups such as the World Federation of Doctors who Respect Human Life, operating on the international level, have been mostly inconsequential.

Abortion has also emerged as a growing problem in many economically developing countries due to their own social and demographic changes. Fertility levels in these countries declined by about one-third between the mid-1960s and the late 1980s from an average of about six children per woman to an average of about four.[82]

The demand for abortion has increased alongside that for smaller family size. This became apparent in Latin America and much of Asia in the 1960s and in several African countries by the early 1990s. These trends are spurred on by a number of socio-economic changes such as urbanization, higher levels of female education and labour force participation. They are also promoted by ideational changes and by the increasing numbers of women in the reproductive age-groups, whose access to and use of effective family planning services remains limited. Nevertheless, governments of nearly all high-fertility countries have come to evince greater concern over population growth and to set up family planning programmes to reduce birth rates. This has in some countries opened up public debate on abortion, a process facilitated at the end of the 1980s by the growing international focus on the health consequences of unsafe abortion.

Several small non-governmental organizations (NGOs) had earlier been working hard to link contraceptive provision with treatment for abortion, and had taken matters further in some instances. The UK-based Marie Stopes International helped introduce menstrual regulation in South Asia. By the early 1990s it had extended its outreach to several East African countries, notably Kenya, and had started to treat complications of unsafe abortion and provide post-abortion family planning services in Sierra Leone. The US-based International Projects Assistance Services (IPAS) completed the development of MVA, a procedure introduced in over 100 countries by 1993, and has sought to reinvigorate attempts to improve post-abortion family planning services.[83] Both organizations have expanded the boundaries of legal interpretations in many countries, as is made clear for Kenya and Mexico. By the end of the 1980s several Dutch, Swedish and Norwegian NGOs, as well as bilateral development agencies, had funded research, advocacy work and treatment for abortion.

The multi-agency-funded International Safe Motherhood Initiative, launched at a major conference in Nairobi in 1987, slowly acknowledged that maternal mortality could not be satisfactorily reduced without confronting unsafe abortion. By the early 1990s the international community of family planning, population and health agencies had convened a number of meetings devoted to the interrelated issues of abortion, unwanted pregnancy and women's reproductive health.[84] This facilitated a process of information sharing, networking and consensus building, sensitizing development agencies to reproductive health care concerns beyond those addressed by conventional family planning programmes. The Ford Foundation approved a ten-year programme to support research on various dimensions of reproductive health.[85] The Population Council, a family planning research organization based in New York, sponsored a limited amount of research on abortion in Kenya and Mexico. In 1995 it completed clinical trials needed for US federal approval of mifepristone, but then suffered a series of setbacks in marketing the preparation. Earlier, President Clinton had lifted abortion-related restrictions in a number of health programmes and reasserted US leadership in the international family planning field. However, legal complications stemming from the political reluctance to deal with the 1973 Helms Amendment to the Foreign Assistance Act (which bars direct US funding for abortion-related purposes overseas) stalled plans by USAID to fund post-abortion family planning services. This led the development agency to modify its newly adopted position that 'reproductive health' includes safe abortion.

More significantly, the political pendulum in the United States swung back in favour of those opposed to the legality of abortion. The Republican Party gained control of the US Congress in late 1994 and its more strident conservatives proposed renewed restrictions on abortion that went beyond the 1973 Helms Amendment. They sought to eliminate USAID and international population assistance on the premise that family planning organizations use such funds to work for the legalization of abortion overseas. By 1996 they succeeded in sharply curtailing US funding for international family planning activities. The Christian Coalition, a political movement made up of Protestant evangelical activists opposed to abortion, strongly backed this agenda. It claimed 1.7 million members in 1,700 chapters across the country and had become a major force in the Republican Party. With anti-abortion groups threatening retribution against any attempts to extend the application of medical methods of pregnancy termination, the manufacturer of mifepristone abandoned the drug and transferred patent rights to one of the pill's developers.[86]

The 1990s have witnessed increased activism over the abortion issue by many organized groups. Conflict was widely apparent before and during the 1994 International Conference on Population and Development, held in Cairo. The UN organized the meeting to approve a twenty-year programme of action setting the course for population programmes. Instead, a bitter dispute over abortion dominated the conference. The US position, which argued that abortion should be safe, legal and rare, reflected the views of the incumbent Democratic administration, its supporters among the 'pro-choice' constituency, and its ideological agreement with women's health advocates, who exerted a major influence on the draft programme of action. The Catholic Church vigorously contested this position, arguing that it promoted global approval of abortion. The abortion debate had moved to the forefront of the world political agenda where it resurfaced – albeit not as emphatically – at the 1995 Fourth World Conference on Women, held in Beijing.

The Cairo conference broadened the approach to reducing world population growth rates by reinforcing the need to empower women through improving their education and health care, as well as through greater social, economic and political equality. It also approved a new international right to reproductive health care, after changes were made to the conference document suggesting that this did not include abortion. The final version of the controversial paragraph 8.25 which dealt with abortion began with the sentence: 'In no case should abortion be promoted as a method of family planning', reflecting the position adopted by the UN meeting a decade earlier in Mexico City. It proceeded to call on governments and private groups to 'deal with the health impact of unsafe abortion as a major public health concern and to reduce the recourse to abortion through expanded and improved family planning services'. Additionally, it recommended that:

> In circumstances in which abortion is not against the law, such abortion should be safe. In all cases, women should have access to quality services for the management of complications arising from abortion. Post-abortion counselling, education and family-planning services should be offered promptly which will also help to avoid repeat abortions.[87]

The Beijing conference built on this carefully crafted compromise that recognized the need to address the problem of unsafe abortions. Delegates went one step further by calling on governments to 'consider reviewing laws containing punitive measures against women who have undergone illegal abortions'. The conference declaration adopted in Beijing also stated that: 'The human rights of women include their right to have control over and decide freely and responsibly on matters related to their sexuality, including sexual and reproductive health, free of coercion, discrimination and violence.' Women's representatives from NGOs in Africa, Latin America and the Caribbean played a more prominent role at this conference than at Cairo, where the controversy over abortion had drowned out their voices and where US women's groups had exercised a strong leadership role. A greater spirit of compromise prevailed at Beijing where the female-headed delegation of the Holy See did not seek to reopen issues that had been decided to the satisfaction of most countries in Cairo. The Clinton administration, wary of domestic criticism and of the upcoming presidential election, softened its stand so that the official US delegation adopted many positions taken by the Vatican, including criticism of coercive abortions and dwelling on motherhood as a role with its own value.

Having presented this overview of key dimensions in the abortion debate, we now turn our attention to describing the design of the study before proceeding to examine these themes in greater depth.

DESIGN OF THE STUDY

This study centres on a detailed comparative examination of abortion debate in three societies, particularly as it pertains to public policy. It explores several aspects of this debate. These include the demography of abortion and its intersection with public health and family planning; the role of data and information in influencing abortion debate and policy; the process by which abortion enters into the public domain, how it is handled in the policymaking process, and with what implications; the way in which debate about abortion policy has evolved and is constructed; and the views, strategies and relative influence of different interest groups, particularly the Catholic Church, in determining abortion discourse and policy.

Abortion practice, debate and policy has not been studied systematically in this way. Rather, researchers have tended to use various frameworks to look at different aspects of induced abortion. Population specialists, for example, might investigate the socio-demographic correlates of abortion and its incidence; legal scholars may examine similarities and differences between abortion laws and construct classification schemes for such purpose; and policy scientists may adopt policymaking models to assess how such laws are formulated. All too often, however, analysts work in one paradigm only or disaggregate the issue of abortion into discrete categories, thereby losing sight of the many critical interrelationships between the various elements of what might be called 'the abortion system'.[88] It is clear that no one central disciplinary framework is suitable for wholesale application to this work that examines the interface of abortion practice, debate and policy. In addition, the comparative perspective here adopted enables the generalizability of hypotheses and theories which, in turn, can be applied to other contexts and make findings more readily comparable. This study has also been designed with a view to providing a benchmark for subsequent research, given that the situation surrounding abortion will be different in the future.

The chapters that follow first set out to clarify demographic estimates of the incidence of abortion and its fertility-inhibiting effects, and appraise the relevant health context in Kenya, Mexico and Poland. This is rendered difficult by severe data limitations due to a lack of societal acceptance of abortion, its illegality in most cases, and poor compliance with reporting procedures even in circumstances where abortion is legal (as in Poland, 1956–93 and 1996–97). For many populations, induced abortion, maternal mortality, and that proportion of such deaths due to abortion, are the most underenumerated demographic indicators. Nevertheless, these empirical realities need to be assessed, because they describe the situation in which abortion takes place and provide arguments to justify policies. The perception and interpretation of these conditions by interest groups, opinion-makers, and decision-making elites may delimit the scope of conflict and of policy alternatives.

The core of the study is based on an interpretative methodology. The author collected field data in Kenya, Mexico and Poland to assess at first hand the context within which abortion is practised, and to identify the beliefs, values, motivations and strategies of important agents and actors engaged in the abortion dispute and seeking to influence abortion policy. The most important primary data source consisted of 162 in-depth, open-ended interviews, each lasting at least one hour. The author conducted these interviews with a comprehensive cross-section of key officials (including government ministers and bishops), activists, influentials, informed observers, as well as health, demographic and family planning experts. In addition, I have examined official and unpublished documents, reports and data, statements, newspaper articles, and interest group iterature, as well as maintained a research diary containing my own field observations. This triangulation of data sources facilitated and strengthened the verification of my findings. The methodology used is explained in more detail in the appendix.

The abortion debate is best understood from a comparative policy-science perspective. This involves the description, analysis and explanation of the formulation and implementation of public policy. In many countries, abortion is increasingly commanding the attention of society as it is identified as a public problem. The issue is also becoming more visible in the political arena and so more likely to be recognized as an agenda item that demands governmental action. Abortion is probably the most divisive public policy issue in the USA. It has come to occupy a similar position in Poland and has the potential to become far more contentious in both Mexico and Kenya. Accordingly, this study makes use of central themes in the conceptualization of the policymaking process as a series of stages of agenda-building. These include agenda-setting, consensus building, elite and community conflict, and issue resolution.[89]

This schema helps illuminate why and how abortion is reaching agenda status, and which policy alternatives are considered. For example, the Polish Communist Party allowed minimal public debate when it altered the law on abortion in 1956; after the regime's downfall, the Catholic Church and its political allies forcefully presented their own position on abortion. This had to compete with a number of diverse policy proposals as resistance grew to the Church's attempt to organize public policy on this and other issues. In Mexico, the Catholic Church and Church-backed groups have so far managed to block attempts by feminists and some reformist politicians to promote a more liberal abortion policy.

The way abortion is considered is influenced by the broader canvas of changing governmental ideologies, shifts in the emphases and strategies of non-governmental actors, systemic changes as have recently occurred in Poland, and profound societal changes like those taking place in Kenya, Mexico and Poland. Such developments may provide both short- and long-term constraints and opportunities for individuals, groups and policymaking elites to alter abortion discourse, policy and practice. Likewise, policymaking and policy implementation are affected by changes in the broader framework of economic, social and political structures within which they occur. This requires an appreciation of such contextual influences as societal pressures, bureaucratic capacities, international conditions, other public policies that impinge on the abortion debate, and the internal dynamics of government.

The majority of writings on family planning and fertility trends and policies have attempted to increase understanding of factors operating at the level of the individual household couple. However, it is opinion-leaders and the decision-making elites that decide on policy, including that concerned with abortion. These influentials may also shape public attitudes and foster a climate conducive to changing public policies. Social scientists have long been analysing the roles elites play in decision-making processes, especially regarding the formulation and implementation of social policies.[90] Elite theory is useful both for the social and political analysis of pluralistic and industrialized societies, and for the study of rapidly changing developing countries where, in most cases, emergent and better-equipped elite cadres are displacing the old, traditional ascribed-status elites, and the role of legislatures in government continues to be minor.

This volume looks at the extent to which abortion policymaking is influenced by elite perceptions of abortion trends, which cannot be so clearly ascertained as fertility trends. More extensively, this analysis examines the demands of interest groups, the perceptions held, the positions adopted, and the strategies used by decision-makers and influentials taking part in the abortion debate. This approach assumes that much of the explanation for the shape of abortion discourse and of the policy process rests on a systematic understanding of their roles and actions. The study further employs insights from group theory and, where appropriate, from organizational theory, to see how collective interests are attempting to influence such processes.

The abortion debate is also a cultural contest between groups characterized by conflicting world views and discourses. The opposing parties in this debate employ rhetorical strategies whose words and ideas carry different meanings. This demands an examination of how abortion debate has evolved and is constructed in different settings since this, too, shapes abortion policy and practice. This is readily apparent, for example, in the USA where conflict over abortion is particularly deep.[91] For example, the terms 'pro-life' and 'pro-choice' are in many ways misnomers. Many among those who profess to be on the side of 'life' downplay the considerations of a pregnant woman, whereas many of those passionately arguing for 'reproductive choice' minimize the nature of foetal life.

WHY KENYA, MEXICO AND POLAND?

Kenya, Mexico and Poland were chosen for fieldwork and detailed study for a number of important reasons. First, in each of these countries, the abortion debate has recently become more heated and is representative of growing conflict over the issue in each region. Second, all are characterized by high abortion rates, reflecting the unmet need for family planning and the reality of contraceptive failure. Third, in all three countries, the Catholic Church commands a significant presence in public life and has more actively opposed legal access to abortion in recent years. The focus on Latin America and sub-Saharan Africa is appropriate, too, given that about 40 per cent of the world's one billion Catholics are Latin Americans and close to 100 million live in Africa, the fastest-growing region of the Church. Poland is mono-ethnic and, like Mexico, mono-religious, although there is a strong anti-clerical tradition in Mexico. Under communism, the Polish church became the focus of national aspirations and of moral fervour. It also gave rise to a pope who has made the protection of unborn life a key concern of his pontificate. Fourth, there is a lack of knowledge about abortion in all these countries (and in neighbouring states) which, if not rectified, may lead to the continuation of misleading accounts and interpretations. Fifth, the international community has been keenly observing developments in all three countries, where changes in governance have enabled groups to make demands which were not possible before. This includes claims to modify abortion policies.

Kenya has long been favoured by Western nations which have viewed it as an African success story. By the late 1980s Kenya also attracted attention for its stalled progress to multiparty democracy. Latin American countries have long looked on Mexico as a pillar of stability in a traditionally unstable region. In the early 1990s the world's media reported widely on the bold economic reforms and the prospect of imminent political change in Mexico, and speculated on what this may mean for the rest of the continent. Despite continued rule by the world's most enduring regime, and renewed economic instability in the mid-1990s, the country remains a crucial symbol of the region's aspirations, which now seem tied to a more open capitalist and pluralist path of development. Poland, meanwhile, caught the world's attention for pioneering more substantive systemic changes. It has been at the forefront of the transformation of East Central Europe from communism to a market economy and a democratic, pluralistic society. It has also been the stage for a major conflict over abortion policy, closely watched in many countries.

At the same time, each of these three countries offers a different regional setting in demographic, cultural and political terms, as well as varying levels of socio-economic development. Table 1.4 presents basic demographic data for all three countries, the estimated gross national product per capita and the human development index. This aggregate socio-economic indicator tracks progress in longevity, education and income, as measured by life expectancy at birth, adult literacy, mean years of schooling, and income, ordered on a scale from 0 to 1. The higher the level, the better. Whereas Kenya has a relatively low rating, Poland and Mexico have quite similar scores on this index, although socio-economic differentials are more marked in Mexico. All three countries command strong links with the advanced capitalist economies but occupy a semi-peripheral or peripheral status in the world political economy.

Birth rates are falling in Kenya where the incidence of abortion is greater than has been assumed to date. Abortion rates may be expected to rise further unless gains in contraceptive use are sustained so as to meet the growing demand for lower fertility. There is evidence of the first stirrings for the liberalization of the restrictive abortion law which Kenya retains from its recent colonial past. Catholic bishops have spoken out against any such move, as they have on issues concerned with more overtly political aspects of public life. The Catholic Church continues to play an important developmental role through the health and education centres it runs.

Mexico has the second largest population in Latin America and the second largest Catholic population, both in the region and in the world. It is at an intermediate stage of fertility decline with abortion illegal but widely practised. In 1990 the Catholic Church successfully mobilized against a liberal abortion measure passed and then suspended by the Chiapas state legislature. Despite growing accommodation between the Church and the national government at the time, Church–state relations are still characterized by many tensions, and abortion remains socially controversial and stigmatized.

Poland is probably the most religious of the three countries as measured by church attendance. Despite the pronatalist orientation of Catholicism, however, the birth rate fell below replacement level in 1989 when there began a number of changes in abortion

Table 1.4   Basic demographic and development indicators for Kenya, Mexico and Poland

Indicator	Kenya	Mexico	Poland
Population 1995 (millions)	27.2	91.8	38.6
Population growth rate, 1990–95 (per cent p.a.)	2.8	1.8	0.1
Total fertility rate (TFR), 1990–95	5.4	3.1	1.9
Life expectancy at birth, 1990–95	56	72	71
Infant mortality rate 1990–95 (per 1,000 live births)	66	34	15
Maternal deaths per 100,000 live births (1990)	650	110	19
Percentage of population under age 15 (1995)	47	36	23
Contraceptive use rate Any methods (per cent)	33	67	75
Modern methods (per cent)	28	57	26
Human development index, 1994	0.463	0.853	0.834
Gross national product, 1995 (US$ per capita)	280	3,320	2,790

Notes: Contraceptive use rates refer to women aged 15–49 in union (be it a formal marriage or a consensual union) and include those whose husbands practise contraception. The data are taken from the most recent reliable survey. For Kenya, they refer to 1993 (Government of Kenya, 1994); for Mexico they refer to 1995 (CONAPO, 1997); for Poland, to 1977.
Modern methods include oral pills, intrauterine devices (IUDs), injectables, sterilization (male and female), condoms, and female barrier methods (diaphragm, foam, jelly, and sponge). Any methods include modern methods and traditional methods (rhythm, withdrawal, abstinence if practised for contraceptive reasons, and folk methods).
The maternal mortality ratios cited are the most recent estimates by the World Health Organization (WHO, 1996). For Kenya and Mexico, they indicate a rough order of magnitude and should not be considered as definitive, as discussed in subsequent chapters.

Sources: UN, *World Population Prospects: The 1996 Revision* (New York: United Nations, forthcoming); UNDP, *Human Development Report 1997*

(New York: Oxford University Press, 1997); World Bank, *World Development Report 1997* (New York: Oxford University Press, 1997); and WHO/UNICEF, *Revised 1990 Estimates of Maternal Mortality: A New Approach by WHO and UNICEF* (Geneva: World Health Organization, 1996).

---

policy, including several shifts in the legal position. Abortion has proved to be one of the most intractable issues for a young democracy undergoing major societal change. Not only has the policy conundrum posed by abortion become more bitterly contested in public than in earlier times, but the ensuing debate is set to remain difficult for a long time to come, as it is in many other countries.

2 Abortion in Kenya: The Tyranny of Silence

Africa occupies a peripheral status in the global political economy, but is not isolated from trends and attitudes spreading from elsewhere in the world. These changes and ideas are altering customs and beginning to promote demand for smaller family sizes. Abortion is likewise being discussed more often for reasons that cannot be explained in terms of indigenous factors alone, even though it had always, to some extent, been practised. Abortion is both a social and a health problem in sub-Saharan Africa (hereafter, Africa), to date largely neglected. This chapter helps fill in some of the knowledge gap, explaining why abortion is emerging as a problem, and why it has still not reached agenda status in Kenya, a country long regarded as a benchmark for a huge continent.

A rise in abortion incidence is taking place in Kenya as birth rates and fertility preferences have started to decline, and contraceptive use, although increasing, remains low. Policymakers have so far been oblivious to the high incidence, mortality and morbidity rates associated with unsafe abortion, its consumption of scarce health-care resources, as well as the serious social problems reflected by these trends. There is now more information in Kenya than elsewhere in Africa to indicate the severity of all these problems, which are being better noticed and can no longer be so easily ignored by a government still unable, if not unwilling, to find a framework for dealing with them. Moreover, debate has recently spilled over from professional circles to society. However, the question of what to do about abortion has not yet been politicized, in so far as few people are willing to take a public stand about it, pressure groups are not actively engaged, and emerging conflict has been largely contained.

Kenya continues to be a locus of international attention. Demographers, for example, have known it as the first African country to adopt a population policy in 1967; for having had the highest recorded natural increase rate in the world (4.1 per cent in the 1970s, a doubling time of 17 years); for one of the most comprehensive data series available for the continent; and for being one

41

of the first African countries to enter the transition to lower fer
tility, holding up the prospect of a new regional model. More ge
nerically, Kenya has been the *enfant cheri* of the West, rather like
Nigeria was before the 1967–70 Biafran War. Its record of politi
cal stability and greater socio-economic progress than elsewhere in
Africa earned the respect of Western leaders, who saw a stable
investment haven, and foreign aid flows to Kenya increased steadily after independence in 1963. The situation began to sour in the
mid-1980s when the one-party state tightened its hold on the parliamentary form of government and became increasingly criticized
for corruption, authoritarianism, and blocking progress towards
democracy. It has presided over growing disparities in income and
wealth, and appointed commissions of inquiry to manufacture consensus about contentious issues that included the deaths of senior
church and public figures.[1] Yet even if no longer a showcase of the
West, Kenya has a large and well-educated elite, remains better
equipped than neighbouring countries, and commands more favourable development prospects.

More than almost any other African country, Kenya is the focus
of a whole system of international networks and coalitions on all
sides of many issues. It has been a preferred location for development specialists, donor organizations, and even two UN specialized agencies – the Centre for Human Settlements (Habitat) and
the Environment Programme (UNEP), the first United Nations body
with headquarters in a developing country. Kenya has hosted major international conferences, such as those to close the UN Decade for Women (in 1985), on Safe Motherhood and on Better Health
for Women and Children through Family Planning (both held in
1987). It has also been the venue of international conferences organized by Catholics opposed to birth control in Africa.

In Kenya as in Africa as a whole, politics has been marked by
the absence of democracy, marginal participation and weak state
structures.[2] Church growth has been rapid, and Africa's importance
to the Catholic Church has grown greatly in turn. By 1995 there
were 100 million African Catholics, up from 15 million in 1955
but, at 14 per cent of the continent's population, probably fewer
than all other Christians and less than the number of Muslims. An
African heads the College of Cardinals that elects the Pope, and
the first Special Synod for Africa was convened in 1994 to examine
the Church's work there. Kenya has one of the continent's highest
national proportions of Christians, about three-quarters of all citi-

zens.[3] The Catholic Church comprises the largest congregation, about one-quarter of all Kenyans, or one in three Christians; the National Council of Churches of Kenya (NCCK) is the mainstream Protestant group whose 35 members include the chief denominations, the Church of the Province of Kenya and the Presbyterian Church of East Africa, which grew out of the Anglican and Scottish church missions, respectively. What these major Christian churches have to say affects many areas of life, including birth control. They have strongly supported civil society and criticized repression. The churches also provide much of the schooling and one-third of all health facilities in rural areas. The efforts made by the medical department of the Kenya Catholic Secretariat (KCS, the national office and executive arm of the bishops) to upgrade its health centres have surpassed those in any other African country. It runs many community-based health care programmes, some 250 health centres and dispensaries, and 30 hospitals, in addition to a family life programme that includes family life education to youth and natural family planning (NFP) instruction for married couples.[4]

The government's family planning programme has long been a sensitive issue due to church opposition, societal preferences for large families, insecurities stemming from ethnic rivalries, fears about the motives of Western aid donors promoting smaller birth rates, and ignorance or misunderstanding about the implications of rapid population growth for social and economic development.[5] The NCCK accepts the need for family planning and has been less vocal over the issue of abortion than the Catholic Church, whose disapproval of family planning has been blunted by the increasing acceptance of such services and, to some extent, transformed into promotion of its own family life programme activities. However, fierce controversy still surrounds the issues of teenage contraception and the content of sex education, and conflict is likely to develop further over abortion. The Catholic Church has protested the increase in immorality that would allegedly result from any measure that would reform abortion policy; but it does not dominate the centre-stage of the abortion debate as in Poland or Mexico.

The increased comment about what was, until only a few years ago, a taboo subject, is concomitant with the rise in incidence and awareness of the problems associated with unsafe abortion. Few have spoken openly about confronting these problems or advocated change in existing policy. This is due to many reasons, such as worries about a backlash, a pervasive fear of polarization over the issue

should it be raised, and the overall very tense political environment. It is commonly perceived that groups will not push the abortion issue unless the government does so first. This contributes to
the neglect of existing problems and confusion as to how they should
be managed. Many do not foresee substantive policy change, but
there are signs that the issue could attain agenda status. For
policymakers, the problem lies in how to accommodate such fears,
misperceptions, actual and potential conflict, along with growing
recognition of the gravity of the situation and the need to do some-
thing about it. However, until concern is translated into greater
policy attention, a tyranny of silence will continue to envelop the
problem of abortion.

ACCESS TO ABORTION SERVICES

The present conservative legal position, accepted from the British
at the time of independence, makes no provision for abortion other
than in the event of a serious threat to a woman's health. This is
in keeping with most African laws on abortion,[6] although in 1996
South Africa – an increasingly important moral, political and economic force on the continent, following its peaceful transition from
a race-based apartheid system to a full participative democracy –
legalised the procedure was legalized for the first 12 weeks of pregnancy.[7] In Kenya, however, following English practice before 1967,
a woman requires two medical opinions and her husband's consent
to obtain an abortion from a gynaecologist, and the threats to both
her physical and mental health need to be justified. The legal position has often been misstated, in large part because the relevant
sections of the penal code are definitionally ambiguous.[8]

While it may still be premature to talk of a lapsed law situation,
the spaces for working within this legal framework are being en-
larged. Abortion services are now more widely available and cov-
ertly advertised, although information on their quality remains difficult
to obtain. Clients might sign a consent form for the 'emergency
evacuation of the retained products of conception', be officially
admitted for a dilatation and curettage (D&C) to treat a gynaecological problem, such as dysfunctional uterine bleeding, or have
their abortion induced in a private clinic and completed as a hospital emergency. Service providers, though sometimes harassed by
police seeking bribes, are unlikely to be investigated unless strongly

condemned in the event of a death. They might then be charged with medical negligence and manslaughter, but not for performing an abortion.

THE MEDICAL DEMOGRAPHY OF ABORTION

In Kenya, the incidence of abortion was first described as a serious public health problem in 1980, but these academic remarks fell on deaf ears.[9] To the extent that plausible data exists, there is general agreement among researchers that the incidence of induced abortion is high and rising, accounting for between 5 per cent and 15 per cent of all births averted by the early 1990s.[10] It is likely that Kenyan abortion rates are higher than in northwestern Europe and comparable to those found in the USA. About 100,000 abortions may have been conducted annually in Kenya during the mid-to-late 1980s, representing some 25 procedures per thousand women of childbearing age. Abortion is estimated to have reduced total potential fertility by about 8 per cent in 1989, a rise from some 3 per cent in 1984.[11]

While there are no data on religious or ethnic differentials, there appear to be no grounds for believing these to be significant. Abortion is probably more common in urban areas, but the author's interviews, discussions and personal observations indicate that it is a problem in rural areas as well. Earlier survey data from the late 1970s suggested that urban and more educated women were increasingly relying on abortion to control fertility.[12] A decade later the 1989 Kenya Demographic and Health Survey (KDHS) showed that more rural than urban women wanted to stop childbearing, because they had on average more children.[13]

Both the incidence and consequences of abortion among adolescents are much higher than is suggested by their proportion in the population. A 1991 survey of youth fertility found that 13 per cent and 28 per cent of young women (mostly aged 15–19) from Nairobi and Mombasa, respectively, had terminated their pregnancies.[14] The author's interviews with gynaecologists and existing reports alike indicate that women hospitalized for abortion at Kenyatta National Hospital (the national teaching and major referral hospital) are predominantly young and single, those least likely to locate and afford safe services, but most likely to be ignorant, fearful and secretive about their unwanted pregnancies. Almost three-quarters are 25 years old or less, an age-group that makes up about half of the female population of childbearing age. The number of cases fluctuates seasonally, with a rise one to two months after school holidays. A study from the late 1980s that included hospital sites outside the capital reported that 46 per cent of abortion patients had between one and three children, 22 per cent had four to six children, and 7 per cent had seven children or more.[15] This suggests that married, multiparous women are increasingly turning to abortion, most likely because of growing socio-economic pressures.

Being pregnant in Kenya is still not only common; it can be quite risky. The maternal mortality rate is estimated to be anywhere from 200 to 650 per 100,000 live births, with marked regional differentials.[16] The higher estimate yields a lifetime risk of maternal death of one in 20. The prevailing opinion among gynaecologists is that abortions poorly performed or carried out in unhygienic conditions account for over one-quarter of these deaths. Between 25 and 40 daily cases of incomplete abortion are treated at Kenyatta National Hospital, or over 10,000 annually, comprising the most frequent diagnosis among gynaecological in-patients and one of the most common of all forms of hospital admissions.[17] In the late 1970s and early 1980s, studies indicated a death rate of about 3 per 1,000 abortion admissions at this hospital; over 60 per cent of acute gynaecological beds tended to be occupied by abortion patients. Over half had sepsis, haemorrhage, or other serious complications, and about one-third returned to the hospital with serious complaints.[18] The introduction of manual vacuum aspiration (MVA) at the end of the 1980s speeded up patient flows and a clinic began to offer post-abortion family planning services in 1992.[19] Some individuals may have extended the use of MVA to induce abortions, although the Ministry of Health has taken steps to ensure that the law is not abused.

Although Kenyatta National Hospital is by far the largest hospital providing for such emergencies, these figures need to be considered in a context where patients prefer to seek services outside the deteriorating formal health sector and where health workers believe they come across a fraction of all abortions. Evacuations are also performed at private hospitals, including the exclusive Aga Khan hospital, and many mission institutions, such as the well-known Chogoria hospital run by the Presbyterian Church in rural Eastern Province. Like Catholic hospitals, these have strict guidelines against abortion but cannot, in good conscience, turn away those who would otherwise die from a poorly performed procedure. Elsewhere, a study of patients at eight hospitals in six provinces in 1988–89 reported a case fatality rate of 6.1 per 1,000 induced abortion admissions. This is over 1,500 times higher than the risk of death (0.4 deaths per 100,000 procedures) then associated with legal abortion in the USA, which has since fallen further.[20]

The current provision of services is inadequate even for the few abortions permitted under the law. Those able to pay, with access to social connections and good information networks, can secure safe operations, unlike many low-income and young women. In late 1991, prices for an abortion in Nairobi ranged from 250 Kenyan shillings (about US$9) charged by 'specialized' women in the deprived area of Eastlands, to as much as 21,000 Kenyan shillings (US$750) charged by one prominent physician. Many urban abortions (and menstrual regulations) are performed in private hospitals, nursing homes and clinics, which derive much of their revenue this way. In rural areas, abortions tend to be performed by paramedics or non-medical people, or are self-induced.

THE RISE OF THE ABORTION QUESTION

The convergence of a number of conditions underlies the increasing incidence and discussion of abortion which, in turn, is giving rise to the question of how this problem should be managed. These include demographic, social and economic pressures, unwanted adolescent fertility, the conflict between traditional and modern influences on families, the modification of cultural and family-centred restraints on sexuality, confusion generated by these and other changes, greater awareness of public health problems, and the increase in research and publicity. These domestic as well as external influences are assessed below.

Domestic influences

Abortion is increasingly contributing to fertility decline now that Kenya is in the midst of fertility transition.[21] In the first three decades since independence, the population almost tripled to 25 million people due to sustained high fertility and falling mortality rates. Almost half of all Kenyans are aged 15 years or less (see Table 1.4). However, the TFR fell from 8.1 births per woman in the late

Table 2.1   Indicators of fertility decline for currently married women
aged 15–49, Kenya

Indicator	1977–78 KFS	1984 KCPS	1989 KDHS	1993 KDHS
Total fertility rate (TFR)	8.1	7.7	6.7	5.4
Mean ideal family size	7.2	6.3	4.8	3.9
Percentage using any family planning method	7.0	17.0	26.9	32.7
Percentage currently using modern contraceptives	6.0	9.7	17.9	27.3
Percentage who want no more children	17.0	32.0	49.4	51.7

Notes: The data refer to the periods 1975–77, 1983–84, 1984–88, and 1990–93 for women aged 15–49, as measured by the Kenya Fertility Survey (KFS) of 1977–78, the 1984 Kenya Contraceptive Prevalence Survey (KCPS), and the 1989 and 1993 Kenya Demographic and Health Surveys (KDHS), respectively. KDHS data for the proportion of currently married women aged 15–49 who want no more children includes sterilized women.

Sources: Government of Kenya, *Kenya Demographic and Health Survey 1989* (Nairobi: National Council for Population and Development, Ministry of Home Affairs and National Heritage; and Columbia, MD: Institute for Resource Development/Macro Systems, 1989); and *Kenya Demographic and Health Survey 1993* (Nairobi: National Council for Population and Development, and Central Bureau of Statistics; and Calverton, MD: Macro International, 1994).

1970s to 5.4 children per woman in the early 1990s (Table 2.1). This sharp fertility decline is due to a rising age at marriage and a near fivefold increase in contraceptive use, from 7 to 33 per cent of currently married women of childbearing age; and a radical shift in favour of modern, more effective methods, which have accounted for nearly all the increase in contraceptive use since 1984. It has been underpinned by a marked shift toward reduced desired family size, down from 7.2 children in the late 1970s to 3.9 children in 1993. Among currently married women aged 15–49, half wanted no more children and one-third of those who were not using contraceptives wanted no more children. Over half of all births in the previous 12 months were reported by their mothers as either mistimed or unwanted, a very high proportion by African standards. These data suggest that much of the unwanted fertility and resort to abortion is due to the unmet need for family planning.

Adolescent sexual activity and unwanted pregnancy are high, whereas contraceptive use is notoriously low and ineffective among youth aged 15–24, who form one-fifth of the population and are its fastest growing component. In 1989 only 2 per cent of women aged 15–19 were currently using modern contraceptive methods, rising to 6.1 per cent in 1993.[22] A higher proportion of people are now exposed to the risk of premarital pregnancies for a greater time-period, because the female age at marriage has risen and the age at menarche has fallen.[23] The total number of pregnancies and abortions will rise as the proportion of women of childbearing age increases and especially as young people continue to initiate sexual activity early, with little knowledge, use or access to contraceptives. Young people do not know who to talk to about avoiding pregnancy, are given contradictory messages by adults, and are ambivalent, misinformed or ignorant about reproductive health.[24]

The confusion over how to deal with these and other trends, the attention given to adolescent fertility, and societal reluctance to sanction access to contraceptives to youth, have made the abortion question more acute and visible. The plight of adolescents with crisis pregnancies is compounded by the low earning capacity of women, the economic crisis, the erosion of family support systems, especially in urban areas, and the lack of adequate social and welfare services. Although the incidence of adolescent pregnancy has not increased, many of these pregnancies now occur outside of marriage and in school. They are also attracting more comment because the expansion of education has greatly increased the opportunity cost of an unwanted pregnancy that can end a schoolgirl's employment prospects in the modern sector. Both society and state have invested heavily in education, which Kenyans have viewed as a ticket to wealth. Inevitably, abortion is increasingly tolerated, if not condoned, where it permits a young woman to continue her studies and prevents her from being trapped in a cycle of poverty, unemployment, marginality and high fertility.

The first estimates of pregnancy-related school drop-out rates received national press coverage, opened up the subject for public discussion, and indicated that there were 10,000 such schoolgirls per year.[25] Publicity about this situation heightens the sense of crisis. As one journalist put it: 'The problem with fertility is that it is difficult to pick up on TFRs. The problem with family planning is that it is not very sexy. But adolescent pregnancy and abortion are both very emotional and easily identified as a big wastage.' In the public mind, this situation has also been linked up with the image of 'sugar daddies', urban men paying school fees and giving gifts to young women in return for sex.

The cultural hostility to fertility control has stemmed from an almost pathological fear of childlessness.[26] Within the last few years, contraception, female sterilization, and abortion have stopped being taboo topics for most people. They are now less sharply contrasted with the virtues of high fertility. This is leading to more discussion and awareness of abortion, as are social changes. Pronatalist values remain firmly rooted but, along with patriarchal structures, are being modified in favour of smaller families and greater decision-making by women.[27] A change regarding women's ideas of what they should get out of their lives is contributing to the incidence of abortion. Ironically, the Catholic Church's stand over birth control may also be leading to higher abortion rates. Some women find it problematic to be seen publicly to procure and use a contraceptive, and then justify its use to their troubled consciences. They are more likely to resort to abortion or to sterilization, a contraceptive method which the Church opposes more strongly than other forms of birth control.

At the 1989 national leaders' conference on population and development, President Moi stated that 'the greatest challenge we face today is for us to influence the attitude of our people towards having smaller families'.[28] Such strong rhetoric opened up debate on population problems and other neglected issues such as abortion, facilitating research efforts and the work of change agents. The Centre for the Study of Adolescence, created in 1988 to secure research funding and provide information about adolescent fertility, soon developed a second focus on abortion.[29] Since the mid-1980s, there has probably been more research on abortion in Kenya than anywhere else in Africa. Even the technical staff of the government's National Council for Population and Development (NCPD, formed in 1982 to coordinate population activities) wanted to estimate the growing incidence of abortion as part of a study to project the components of fertility decline.[30] The Council itself is unlikely to address the issue more formally because its board comprises government officials and permanent secretaries (political appointees) who would not pursue the matter without higher authority for fear of being dismissed.

The growth in research interest coincided with rising awareness of health issues generally, with more information read by a better educated citizenry. As one researcher remarked to the author: 'In our own small way, we are making the topic more discussable to the point that journalists are coming to talk about it with us, even though we are still only scratching the surface.' In the process, the problem of coordinating research and policy has come increasingly to the fore.

External influences

In spite of the US 'Mexico City policy' curtailing funds for abortion research, several external funding agencies became supportive of work on maternal mortality, adolescent fertility, and abortion. Problems in these areas were highlighted by the international conferences on the situation of women held in Nairobi in the mid-1980s. The Population Council recognized the need to promote a broader examination of abortion. With grant monies from the Swedish International Development Agency, it supported research that included the first community-based study to document the widespread incidence of abortion not recorded by hospital-based data.[31] Two external change agents, IPAS (International Projects Assistance Services) and Marie Stopes Kenya, helped introduce MVA equipment. Marie Stopes Kenya also began providing a broad range of reproductive health services, including menstrual regulation, through its expanding clinic network.

Although Kenya's strong ties with Western countries have become strained politically – due to domestic and external criticism of President Moi's autocratic style, worsening human rights record, and economic mismanagement – they have been strengthened in other areas. Nairobi is a centre for over 100 foreign journalists reporting on Africa. Kenyans are now exposed to international coverage of the abortion issue. Television pictures of street demonstrations and pickets outside US abortion clinics may affect public discourse and the assumptions of policymakers, who have also had to take stock of the changes in USAID funding of population aid programmes. Local journalists are beginning their own analyses of abortion consistent with international concerns, the growing number of local studies looking into these issues, and increasing public comment on the topic.

Western influences can be discerned in the discourses raised over abortion, particularly by religious groups, women and journalists. The terms 'abortionist', 'pro-choice', and 'pro-life' are increasingly heard in Kenya although, for historical reasons, external influences are not openly admitted to and can be negatively perceived. This is why those seeking to reform abortion policy believe they must generate debate domestically for their cause to become widely accepted. They have also attempted to shape debate in terms of the individual woman, and especially the adolescent faced with the problem pregnancy, rather than employ labels that refer to onlookers with rigid views on her situation.

THE CONDUCT OF THE ABORTION DEBATE

Public debate on abortion has been episodic but controversial. For example, in 1979–80 Catholic bishops responded strongly to a perceived attempt to legalize abortion, when the new government began to increase its commitment to family planning. Parliamentarians were then told: 'Nothing would more effectively destroy the moral fabric of our people than would legalized abortion.'[32] In a pastoral letter, the bishops referred to abortion as 'the most radical method of birth prevention, and one which deserves the most serious and forthright condemnation'.[33] They restated their support for maintaining a restrictive abortion law at a meeting with President Moi and through a specially convened 'pro-life working group', which also recommended that they start a family life programme to address the concerns of families, including natural family planning (NFP) and family life education for youth.[34]

Catholic bishops vigorously attacked family planning and abortion about the time of the 1984 national leaders' conference and the World Population Conference in Mexico, and before the Pope visited Nairobi at the end of the 1985 Eucharistic Congress on the Family. The head of the Kenyan Church cautioned those advocating birth control and abortion were working against the will of God; his comments had to be clarified by his secretariat.[35] At the 1985 UN Women's Decade conference and the accompanying NGO Forum, several Western 'right-to-life' groups voiced their opposition to abortion, 'artificial' contraception, and the IPPF.[36] The Catholic Church restated that abortion was not an acceptable method of birth control at the 1989 national leaders' seminar. On the eve of the 1994 UN Conference on Population and Development, Catholic bishops from across East Africa and the Philippines met in Nairobi to condemn abortion, as well as sex education and the use of contraceptives by youth.[37]

Only some senior public officials have publicly advocated policy change, and their calls have not been followed up. An outspoken former director of the Ministry of Health's Division of Family Health reportedly appealed several times for the legal provision of abortion services on health grounds, and to legitimize a widely known common act.[38] In 1991 the Kenya Law Reform Commission, a body which formulates prospective laws for parliament, indicated that the existing law may be obsolete and recommended that abortion be legally permitted in rape cases.[39] The chief government adviser on health matters recognized abortion as a public health problem, stressed the need to improve post-abortion family planning services, and invited the medical profession to draw up new recommendations on who should be able to procure an abortion so that he could pass these on to government. This was a clear call for greater acceptance of the need to protect the health of pregnant women in all dimensions, if not an endorsement for deregulating abortion services as such.[40] The official did not remain in his post long enough, however, for the guidelines to reach him.

Abortion has been raised peripherally in the context of discussion of children's rights. In an appeal to the Presidential Task Force on Child Law, a district probation officer argued that the restrictive abortion law serves no useful purpose, is ineffective in preventing abortion, and should be abolished because 'the crime of abortion had no complainants' and its 'only victims were pregnant women, who agreed to the abortion on a contractual basis with those helping them to abort'.[41] Although it is unclear whether this was a move to test the waters for reform, the NCCK promptly issued a statement guarding against any such measure. Such calls reflected the indirect process by which the government had earlier brought up the subject of contraceptive social marketing.[42]

Debate has started on abortion, a topic which used to be largely unmentionable. It has yet to reach a mature stage but, as it develops, positions are likely to become clearer and less cryptic. The evolution of abortion debate may follow an incremental process similar to that on family planning. Everyone is now prepared to discuss this, unlike earlier, and debate has moved on from contraception and the spacing of families to adolescent fertility. At the first Inter-African Conference on Adolescent Health (held in Nairobi, 1992), Kenya's Vice-President described reproductive health concerns as 'one of the most serious challenges facing African policymakers today'.[43] The meeting launched the African Association for the Promotion of Adolescent Health and proposed re-examination of the legal impediments to abortion, related care and treatment.

The impetus for debate comes from medical practitioners who have to deal with abortion, as well as from elite women and higher socio-economic groups. It also arises from increased societal concern over adolescent fertility, fuelled by recent studies indicating the high incidence and cost of abortion in society; and from external influences. While there is little consensus on how to deal with abortion, there is growing recognition that a problem exists, especially among adolescents. The government is beginning to acknowledge that this situation cannot continue indefinitely, not least because of the human costs and the economic waste it entails. At the same time, the Catholic Church and the NCCK have spoken out against any attempts to initiate policy reform. The debate that is taking place is elitist, dispersed, and at a very fluid stage. Lobbying is quietly occurring at workshops and such fora, typically behind closed doors, but there is no consolidated effort to effect change. A full-scale debate has yet to be launched by medical, women's or other groups.

Among professional groups, the discourse largely reflects the interests and findings of researchers. These include health concerns, unwanted adolescent pregnancy, the widespread incidence of abortion despite its legal prohibition and, more quietly and obliquely, the prospect that the state itself considers the law anachronistic. Medical professionals could have the greatest input in abortion debate, but physicians have not engaged in a dialogue with policymakers. They are only raising the issue in a very small way, with one prominent advocate described to the author as 'a lone voice in the wilderness'.

Public discussion of abortion tends to be poorly informed and meshed in moralistic overtones, as illustrated by the mostly polemical letters that have been published in the press. Debate has barely touched on legal or rights considerations. The discourse of tradition is a recurrent theme, underlining that abortion is part of a broader struggle over the places of tradition and of women in a modernizing nation. In the past, abortion was regarded as a woman's 'misfortune' or folly, but traditionalists (including elders and religious leaders, notably from the Catholic Church) tend to frame abortion as a moral issue and command political influence. Indeed, ethnic groups, courts, churches and the government have all played on recent historical dislocations to manipulate the theme and language of tradition for different ends.[44] One such purpose has been to undervalue and marginalize women's public roles and to champion their roles as wives or mothers, rather than risk claims to political power. Reformers are somewhat divided between wanting to cast debate in social, health or legal terms, and are unsure how to use political channels to do so.

There are signs that attitudes may be changing as more people hear about and are affected by abortion more closely than before, as the attendant problems of street children and unwanted childbirth have become more visible, and as other former taboos, such as child abuse and violence against women, are increasingly discussed. Few think of abortion as a women's rights issue, however, and women's groups have not extended their claims to the abortion issue. Although debate has converged on health aspects and reflected discussion of adolescent pregnancy, it is still rather general, without a specific focus, and with a heavy religious-moral overlay. This view of abortion as immoral and criminal remains the basis of the controversy and is reinforced by the body politic, suggesting a political expediency in maintaining the status quo.

THE KENYAN CATHOLIC CHURCH AND THE ABORTION QUESTION

Although the role of the state remains paramount in determining policy issues in Kenya, other actors may exert leverage in policymaking. These include religious leaders, physicians and other health care providers, women's and family planning groups, researchers and change agents. The churches make up the most significant force with which the state has to contend. It is the Catholic Church which has had the most to say about birth control, is poised to resist strongly abortion policy reform efforts, and is the major organizational group investigated in this study.

The importance of the Kenyan Church to Catholicism was underscored when it hosted in 1985 the first ever Eucharistic Congress on African soil, closed out by Pope John Paul II. It remains organizationally tied to Rome, the upholder of doctrine and identity, but has moved to greater self-determination and localization.[45] The Church's leadership has been 'africanized' and Nairobi has developed into an international training centre for theological studies.

Church–state relations and birth control

The Catholic Church in Kenya is highly respected due to its inner unity, dignified leadership and strong involvement in nation-building and development. Papal visits in 1980, 1985 and 1995 heightened the profile of a Church that commands a significant influence in public life. Mwai Kibaki, the accomplished Catholic former vice-president who frequently championed the cause of family planning, stated when in office that 'politics and religion are inseparable'.[46] Kenyan bishops have wryly observed that both Presidents Kenyatta and Moi called their churches the consciences and watchdogs of society.[47] Both presidents have sought to keep a good *modus vivendi* with the churches because of their numerical strength, authority and valued role in health care; but they have also been suspicious of their independent status and have tended to see the churches as serving the state. Not wanting to be used by dominant groups, Catholic leaders have preferred to raise their voice only on what they see as religious or moral issues, including birth control, and adopted a low-key political stance until the late 1980s.

Both church and state have found it difficult to reconcile their differences over birth control. Recent conflicts show that the government remains susceptible to church pressure. This is significant because controversy and debate over family planning are important precursors to those on abortion and are in many ways integral to it. In 1988 the Catholic Church organized a petition drive and 'warned' against staging a scheduled symposium on adolescent sexuality and fertility. President Moi called off the meeting shortly before it was to open.[48] With the NCCK, the Church successfully mobilized against government plans to promote contraceptive social marketing. In 1989, 1993, 1994 and 1997 it put off governmental implementation of a family life education curriculum (which included family planning information and education) in schools.[49] Several informants pointed out that these issues were discussed at the NCPD's general council, where influential civil servants expressed concern that the Catholic Church's pressure had led the government to prohibit contraceptives for the young and unmarried.

The Church has been instrumental in thwarting plans to promote condoms as an AIDS prevention measure. This is particularly problematic because of the gravity of the AIDS (acquired immunodeficiency syndrome) crisis, a situation compounded by low use of condoms, their identification with prostitutes, and the high prevalence of sexually transmitted diseases (STDs) which channel HIV infection.[50] However, there are limits to church engagement in debate about family planning, which the state has occasionally used as a litmus test for deciding who is loyal to the government. Having secured a seat on the NCPD, funds for natural family planning (NFP), and being consulted by the government which recognizes its positive efforts on 'family life', the Catholic Church cannot oppose contraceptive use more strongly. It has also been influenced by the spirit of cooperation and 'harambee' that has generally prevailed between the state, the churches and ethnic groups.[51]

The Church and abortion

Catholic bishops do not want to enter into a public dispute over abortion. They believe the issue is best handled at the local level within their pastoral programmes, including family life. They are content that their institutional stand on abortion is well known and, unlike the case with contraceptives, supported by the present legal position and probably by most Protestant churches. They are unlikely to address the issue very forcefully unless there is a clear attempt to legalize abortion. The Secretary General of the Episcopal Conference informed the author that the bishops feel there may be such a move 'under the umbrella of concern about the situation at Kenyatta National Hospital'.[52] The bishops' spokesman also stated that 'controlling population growth is all tied up with abortion' and that the turbulent political equation has distracted the bishops from preparing a pastoral letter on this and other family life issues. The bishops derive their information on the abortion situation from diocesan family life workers, Catholic hospitals (which tend not to attract abortion cases) and, at least in some instances, an awareness of the data from the Kenyatta National Hospital. There is, nonetheless, a perception even among devout Catholics that while some bishops realize that abortion is not just a moral, theological or philosophical issue, most are far removed from the problem and their perceptions may be overly based on confessions they have heard and on anecdotal reports.

Catholic leaders do not see any reason to change existing policies on abortion. They consider the growing numbers of street children to be primarily a socio-economic problem, connected with the allocation of resources. They explain the high incidence of abortion in Nairobi as a product of urban dislocation. Some orthodox

Catholics consider that 'abortion is all business for physicians'. Others recognize that they cannot resent those who are saving women's lives from botched abortions, even if they think that many physicians have an indifferent attitude and a conflict of interest over abortion.

The family planning debate and the question of population growth have had an impact on the Catholic Church. The hierarchy has been influenced by the initiatives of lay Catholics, the needs to support Church teaching on marriage and to counter charges that it was not helping couples plan their families. Church authorities acknowledge 'a big change in church thinking on family life issues' and have increasingly focused on promoting family life education in schools and NFP instruction in church health centres and parishes.[53] This has been achieved with the aid of the Family Life Counselling Association of Kenya, a lay Catholic group formed in 1977 that receives support from the bishops but operates outside their direct control. However, it has proved more difficult to constitute a Catholic medical association that would encourage adoption of NFP and an orthodox Catholic viewpoint on abortion. Moreover, despite having much to say about protecting life and maintaining that unwanted pregnancy can be prevented through value-oriented education, abstinence and (in the case of married couples) NFP, the bishops have paid little attention to alternatives to abortion.

Others within the Church began to do so in the 1980s. In Nairobi Catholic sisters opened a centre to help single mothers and to seek adoption for those unable to keep their babies. A second centre was founded by a Marianist brother to provide a socio-economic alternative through basic job training (in dressmaking, sweatermaking and bookbinding) for poor, young women considering abortion.[54] For some, it performs a useful function; to critics, it is just another 'band aid' that perpetuates the dependency of young women.

Although the bishops lack resources to run such institutions, their existence has enabled churchmen to talk more openly about unwanted pregnancy and single parenthood. Until now the Church's whole world view was based on the pretence that such things did not happen and that talking about them would somehow promote single motherhood. Other churchmen piously claimed that the problem had to be solved sooner and stressed the need for premarital chastity. The problem itself was less common in the past, when extended family structures were more able to provide support. However, the Catholic Church has focused its concern more on teenage sexual activity than a global look at its causes and consequences. It has historically contributed much to improving the position of African women, particularly through the provision of education, but Church leaders show little new thinking on how to enhance this further. Even sympathetic observers described the Catholic Women's Association to the author as 'practically defunct' and 'quite dormant on everything'.

The perceived need to strengthen dispersed efforts against a possible push to legalize abortion led to the formation of 'Friends for Life' in 1991. This small, informal, and predominantly Catholic group has criticized calls made to legal bodies to change abortion policy. Its weekly counselling round at the Kenyatta National Hospital earned the trust of Caritas (Catholic) nurses working at the hospital, but caused friction with overburdened physicians and nurses opposed to activities that may cause offence and harassment to patients, particularly those with 'inevitable' or 'incomplete' abortions.[55]

Opponents of a more liberal abortion regime have resorted to several different rhetorical strategies. They have appealed for the protection of moral and spiritual values as part of an African heritage that keeps African families strong and stable. A common refrain is that: 'the abortionists' campaign for introduction of permissive abortion law in Kenya has been going on in parallel with the promotion of contraception and population control'.[56] The Pope himself has come close to suggesting similar sentiments. When addressing a huge crowd in the presence of President Moi and his senior ministers in Nairobi, he effectively equated abortion and contraception by declaring: 'anti-life actions such as contraception and abortion are wrong and are unworthy of good husbands and wives'.[57] Demographic, public health and scientific evidence has been misread, misunderstood and misused. A memorandum on the draft 1994 Cairo conference document alleged that the meeting's hidden agenda included the destruction of family life and called on the faithful to show their opposition by signing the memorandum. The Vice-President who led the official Kenyan delegation promised national religious leaders that the government would support neither the legalization of abortion (except in the case of saving the life of the pregnant woman) nor the use of contraceptives by young children. Not satisfied with his remarks, the Kenyan Catholic Church sent its own delegation to attend the meeting and present its views and concerns.[58]

External linkages

Although some churches have incorporated views on abortion held by their overseas parent churches, there has been no sustained movement of 'pro-life' activists from the USA, be they Catholic or Protestant. Nevertheless, the author's extensive interviews and discussions with clergy members, officials of the Kenya Catholic Secretariat (KCS), and informed observers show that the Catholic Church's position has been buttressed by its international connections.

Non-Kenyan nationals are actively engaged in the work of the KCS's Medical Department, although some of the more extreme views held by foreign missionaries have been inconsequential.[59] The controversial US film *The Silent Scream* is shown and a similar film (*Your Crisis Pregnancy*) has been made in the Kiswahili language. There have been only sparse contacts with the International Right-to-Life Federation (linked to the US-based National Right-to-Life Committee) in Rome, although a Kenyan priest once served on its steering committee and the federation supports a local affiliate in Zambia. Human Life International has an office in Zambia and its director has visited Kenya, but it is not active in Kenya probably because abortion is legally restricted, the Church has a better developed family life programme than elsewhere in the region, and Human Life International is more interested in lobbying activities. KCS representatives stated that they receive publications from this group and information from the Vatican and the International Federation for Family Life Promotion on moves to change abortion laws in other countries. The Washington-based federation has assisted Kenyan Church groups in promoting NFP, especially the Billings method. Other information is received and exchanged through interpersonal contacts, as at the three international Catholic conferences held in Nairobi in the 1980s.

Of these, the fourth PLAN (Protect Life in All Nations) congress was timed to coincide with the UN Women's Decade meetings to lobby women's leaders. Delegates sent letters to the Pope and President Moi, condemned the UN Convention on the Elimination of all Forms of Discrimination for its 'anti-family ideology', and urged the World Union of Catholic Women's Organizations to withdraw its support from it. The conference resolved to form a pan-African pro-life movement with a separate Kenyan chapter and criticized the USA for funding family planning programmes which led to abortions,[60] although the Reagan administration had already begun to curtail funds for family planning on such a premise. Many who attended the conference judged it favourably at the time, but there was no follow-up, probably due to a 'lack of initiative' and the difficulty of sustaining motivation.

In 1989 the publicity surrounding the fifth congress of the International Federation for Family Life Promotion was likewise not capitalized upon. Speakers again denounced abortion but, in accordance with the conference theme of 'Health and child spacing through natural family planning and family life education', mostly dwelt on the positive aspects of NFP. These were stressed by President Moi who opened the conference attended by some 400 participants from 81 countries. However, those promoting NFP and family life education with a strong moralistic orientation still do not have one voice.

At the 1985 International Eucharistic Congress and on his other visits to Kenya, John Paul II has reiterated the Vatican's position on all matters of birth control, including abortion, and reinforced the local church's presence in public life. He has reminded local bishops that they should not be quiet on these issues. The Papal Nuncio, the representative of the Holy See who has generally assumed a low profile in Kenyan matters, closed out the PLAN Congress by declaring:

> The Church would like to see strong pro-life movements particularly in the developing world where the proponents of birth control have directed all their energies. I am happy here in Kenya the pro-life group is developing fast and I promise it any possible assistance so that it can be a good example in Africa.[61]

It is unclear what tension, if any, exists between Rome and Kenyan bishops, who publicly continue to present a united front and who have restated the Pontiff's stress on family life, the value of NFP, disapproval of contraceptives and strong condemnation of abortion. The first Synod of African Bishops held in Rome in 1994 assailed the 'individualistic and permissive culture which liberalizes abortion and makes of the death of the child simply a matter for the decision of the mother'. However, the issues of priestly celibacy and traditional marriages apparently received greater attention.[62]

In general, educated Catholics who hold key positions in public life have not played an active role in debate about abortion. At the same time there have been sufficient devout Catholics holding posts in various ministries to disrupt the state's efforts to implement family planning education, and who are likely to upset attempts to ease restrictions on abortion services. The conservative order Opus Dei has a small presence in Kenya and appeals to that sector which wants a strong, authoritative voice. Others consider it reactionary on most issues; indeed, throughout the 1980s, KCS staff watched carefully to ensure that it would not exert influence on their family life programme.[63]

The position of non-Catholic religious groups

It is difficult to establish the position of the many Protestant churches which lack the central authority found in the Catholic Church. They have left it to the NCCK to pronounce on abortion, which strongly rejected abortion as a birth control measure in its first major statement on the topic prepared in late 1991.[64] The Christian Health Association of Kenya (an executive arm of the NCCK that is essentially quite autonomous in its operations) offers family planning services through about 200 health facilities, but has never issued a statement on abortion. Its official position cannot differ from that of its member churches, which may cover a range of views even if they nominally maintain a public front against abortion. Of the larger NCCK members, the Church of the Province of Kenya, the Presbyterian Church of East Africa, and the Methodist Church actively support family planning, preach on the need to plan families carefully, and look on unwanted pregnancy more leniently than does the Catholic Church.

Many small evangelical Protestant missions have recently arrived from the USA and have sharpened denominational competition in Kenya. The support from US evangelical churches has enabled Crisis Pregnancy Ministries to start counselling services for young Nairobi women. The group perceives a vacuum for its work and is seeking to expand in Kenya and elsewhere in Africa, modelling its services on the extensive network of affiliated Crisis Pregnancy Centers in the USA and Canada set up by the Christian Action Council.[65] It attempts to redress a young woman's problems in terms of counselling and the provision of maternity and infant clothes; but with young Kenyan women having little autonomy, keeping an unwanted pregnancy may not be an acceptable alternative on social, economic, health or other grounds.

Kenya's Islamic minority accounts for no more than 6 per cent of Kenyans, is concentrated in the coastal region, and, like adherents of traditional religions, is limited in its significance to policy-making. Although Muslim leaders have accepted all contraceptive methods except sterilization, they have shown little interest in promoting family planning and are widely perceived to skirt around the issue of abortion. Their reluctance to discuss the topic in detail with the author even seemed to exceed Catholic sensitivities.

THE ROLE OF OTHER ACTORS: A CASE OF STUDIED NEGLECT

There are many reasons why the abortion debate in Kenya is marked by the absence of clearly defined pressure groups advocating policy reform.[66] Some of these reasons are common to all groups, as explained below, while those specific to women's groups, the medical profession, family planning agencies and several external change agents are clarified afterwards.

Many groups, including the government, fear antagonizing elders, traditionalists, and the churches over this issue. In particular, the Catholic Church has talked most dismissively of teen pregnancy, promiscuity and abortion, often seemingly in one breath. No one wants to be accused of promoting what is illegal, morally complex, and politically awkward. The authoritarian state and the deteriorating political situation have made people wary of pushing issues, unless there is a guarantee at the highest level that change can be affected. The lack of political participation is compounded by internal divisions, minimal institutional coordination, and a lack of understanding about how to open up discussion and influence policymakers.

Medical, women's and family planning groups are all divided, both among themselves and over abortion, making it difficult to work on a common objective. Whereas some family planning groups, for example, think of abortion as a back-up to contraception, others are more reserved. Networking and coalition-building is discouraged by institutional jealousies and a political system that has sought to limit associational life. In the volatile political climate, cooperation with external groups over controversial issues runs the risk of being stymied as working for 'foreign masters'. Transnational linkages between women's groups have been impeded by the perceived arrogance and ethnocentrism of at least some Western feminists. Similarly, there has been friction between Kenyan and overseas-based Catholic groups.[67]

Physicians could present a cogent case for abortion policy reform because they are least likely to be deemed subversive by the state, command international connections, and are highly respected. Until 1994, however, they had not even used their prestige and influence to improve their own conditions,[68] underscoring their limited political insight and reflecting the lack of a well-defined history of a labour movement in Kenya. Similarly, women have not played an important role in fighting for their rights and asserting themselves, which is what abortion law reform demands.

Like physicians, the family planning community is made up of technocrats who can advise, but not necessarily convince policymakers. Physicians, who are more valued, are seen as neither particularly effective nor vocal in their advisory role on health and medical matters. They neither know how to explain technical arguments in a simple way, nor how to influence policy elites whose views on abortion are hard to discern. It is unclear how far politicians can be pushed on this matter and how they can be convinced of its saliency. NGOs in general do not know how to promote the issue, the limits to which are imposed by cultural and social constraints, as well as political parameters. Lawyers themselves have expressed no interest in the abortion issue, despite being more cognizant than others of the non-native origins and non-enforcement of current legal prohibitions on abortion.

Women's groups

At least one academic authority has castigated women's leaders for being careerist, weakly committed, and playing to the tune of the patriarchal system.[69] Their failure to lobby more ably for change indicates a lack of effective and visible leadership. This is true even after allowing for the gender inhibitions and institutionalized discrimination which impede women's leaders from more clearly articulating their positions, but which can also quickly become a rationalization for a lack of action. Women remain grossly underrepresented in parliament and within the ruling party hierarchy; however, there are now enough female lawyers and magistrates in strategic positions to examine defective, discriminatory or unimplemented laws.

The 'Kizito tragedy' highlighted the inability of women's groups to make a political impact. Rampaging boys killed 19 girls by suffocation, sexually assaulted 71 others, and injured 64 more at a school ironically named after the African patron saint of children, St. Kizito. The deputy principal of the school stated: 'the boys meant no harm, they only wanted to rape'.[70] Women's leaders condemned the violence, but failed to sensitize the public further on gender issues and to insist on stronger policy initiatives over gender equity and violence against women. This is why many social commentators feel that women's groups lack a clear, goal-oriented programme and are essentially responding to the conditional needs of the moment.

There are other barriers to women's mobilization in support of legal access to abortion. Despite many initiatives to improve the status of women, traditional attitudes and many laws still act against them and, ironically, women remain marginalized in the country that hosted the UN's Women's Decade Conference.[71] The lack of an organized feminist community hinders attempts to promote women's rights. There are many women's groups, but they tend to be weak or unrepresentative, structurally and geographically isolated. Most exclude the young and the poor and there are deep divisions between elite women who run these groups and those they claim to serve. Whereas well-educated women may talk forcefully about women's rights, few women will do so in rural areas. The lack of sensitivity and awareness of women's leaders to abortion is tied up with a general indifference and class bias, since better-off women have access to good quality services. They may also perceive other issues to be more urgent and achievable in the short term.

Maendeleo ya Wanawake ('Progress for women'), by far the largest grassroots women's organization, will not take on sensitive, contentious matters and has been widely dismissed as a political sham since it was coopted by the state in the mid-1980s.[72] Its conservative leadership has been staffed by senior political appointees, eschews feminist rhetoric and has acted to disempower more activist women's organizations. These have included the Greenbelt Movement whose outspoken leader, probably Africa's best-known environmentalist, has aptly stated: 'women who are within government see it as a privilege to be among men and therefore do not want to rock the boat'.[73] Several disenchanted women's leaders and academics told the author: 'Kanu-Maendeleo does nothing because it is part of the system' and 'the government interferes; it is the one that dictates and structures the issues'. The state's Women's Bureau is ineffective, poorly funded, and still less likely to discuss abortion.

The medical profession

Some gynaecologists who know well the scale of existing problems at the Kenyatta National Hospital and elsewhere have taken the lead in attempting to influence debate about abortion. They have concluded that it is incumbent on their profession to advance this issue and to ensure that women's groups and others have the requisite information to do so. However, many more physicians favour providing abortions discretely rather than pushing for legislative change, risk unleashing hostilities and perhaps being marginalized in the process. Most will not press for reform because it is not in their financial interest.[74]

Medical bodies are unlikely to take up the matter in the near future given their conservative nature and failure to convey sufficient concern over this and other public health problems.[75] The Kenya Medical Association (KMA) is said to favour improved access to abortion services on health grounds, but neither wants abortion to be treated as a family planning method, nor for it to be legalized unless services are well organized.[76] Some government health officials have regarded the Kenya Obstetrics and Gynaecological Society as a pressure group for abortion.[77] Like the KMA, however, it lacks a tradition of lobbying, has not forcefully presented its resolutions to policymakers, and many of its members hold a financial stake in the present situation and do not see abortion as their problem.

The Kenya Medical Women's Association has achieved far better publicity. With the Medical Women's International Association, it organized a regional conference on safe motherhood in 1993 and has advised the Ministry of Health on the subject. However, it has been conspicuously silent about abortion, deferring to the KMA to adopt a position.[78] Yet, as one observer noted, who praised the head of the Kenya Medical Women's Association as a convincing educator and a highly competent professional, 'what is safe motherhood without the option of safe abortion?'[79] Clearly, the organization does not seek to confront what could be controversial: like other groups, it will only move on an issue incrementally and opportunistically should the issue become important to it.

Family planning groups

The social conservatism extends to family planning agencies, which have assumed a low profile in debate about abortion. Some have started to provide post-abortion contraceptive counselling, but all remain cagey about mentioning the 'A-word'. As with other groups, they evince a fear of unknown forces that is not altogether justified. Nevertheless, it has proved very difficult to establish and improve family planning services which are only now being accepted for unmarried people, and only nominally for their public health rationale. This has impeded the development of reproductive health services. Providing abortion, if legally permitted, would also mean diverting resources from family planning.

External constraints, such as the 'Mexico City policy', have precluded abortion-related activities. The programme of the Family Planning Association of Kenya (the largest NGO providing family planning services) is tied to the mission statement of IPPF, its parent donor. The IPPF's mandate focuses on enabling women and couples to better manage the number, spacing and timing of their children; until 1995 it did not advocate access to safe, legal abortion services in the event of an unwanted pregnancy. On the eve of the 1994 Cairo conference, delegates of IPPF member affiliates from 20 African countries accepted the 'Mauritius Declaration'.[80] This urged governments to reduce unwanted pregnancies and unsafe abortions through strengthening family planning services, providing better emergency treatment for incomplete abortion, working towards a more liberal legal interpretation, and increasing awareness of the costs of unsafe abortion. However, the Family Planning Association of Kenya's management committee includes politicians who may have their own reservations about abortion. Senior staff members acknowledged to the author the need to present existing abortion problems more forcefully to policymakers, but stressed they must first 'step in safe water', pointing to the difficulties faced in setting up youth counselling centres in Nairobi and Mombasa.

External change agents

In the late 1980s, several policy entrepreneurs began quietly but significantly to shift the parameters of abortion debate. Whereas the Population Council and the Centre for the Study of Adolescence promoted research, IPAS (International Projects Assistance Services) and Marie Stopes Kenya sought to negotiate improved abortion care. IPAS helped extend to all district hospitals the use of manual vacuum aspiration (MVA) for treating incomplete abortions. By 1992 three Protestant mission hospitals had also begun to use MVA, and IPAS had commenced work in five other African countries.[81] Within five years of opening its first African clinic in a poor area of Nairobi in 1986, Marie Stopes Kenya operated eight clinics in Kenya, planned ten more, and had expanded into other African countries. These offer menstrual regulation and a broad range of reproductive health services which are subsidized for low income women. Its staff believe they have not encountered problems because their organization is seen as a well managed, non-profit operation that provides jobs, respects the law by not advertising its services, and is making a positive impact on several major health problems. This includes improving AIDS awareness, treating STDs and other illnesses, providing contraceptive services and reducing rapid population growth.[82]

BARRIERS TO REFORMING ABORTION POLICY

Despite the growing awareness, discussion and research about abortion, official recognition that it demands policy attention is still lacking. This neglect is due not only to the position of the Catholic Church and the lack of activity over the issue by women's, medical, and family planning groups. It also results from socio-cultural norms and public ideas, particularly on the role of women; the confusion over how best to handle this issue, as with the disruption of sexual and reproductive norms in general; the inertia stemming from the existing situation; and competition for scarce resources from other important health issues, most recently including AIDS. Tense church–state relations and various political considerations pose additional barriers to reforming abortion policy. These obstacles are examined below.

Socio-cultural norms and public ideas play an important role in determining abortion policy by including particular interests and excluding others. On this matter, they are reinforced by a powerful symbiotic relationship between the Catholic Church (as well as other religious bodies) and the traditionalists who wield considerable power among policymakers. Abortion is said to be against cultural traditions and societal values; it is held to be an irresponsible, if not a criminal behaviour, which should be averted by all means. The abortion issue is implicitly defined in line with widely shared public ideas pertaining to traditional social roles of women. Underlying such views are fixed attitudes that do not allow for individual circumstances and which belie an excessive focus on the moral situation of women, not simply the morality of abortion *per se*. They reflect the concerns voiced about making contraceptives available to teenagers and, earlier, to married women, which have focused on the alleged corrupting effects of contraceptives on the morality of those using them. In a similar vein, feminism is dismissed as foreign and divisive, threatening to African nationalism and to the tradition of the woman as homemaker.

This helps explain why the colonial origins of the current legal position on abortion have not become an issue; why everyone is wary of advocating, or even opening up, discussion about abortion; and why policymakers are cautious about proposing policies that may seem unacceptable, despite the cultural, social and behavioural changes that have occurred. Even women's leaders are influenced by religion, customs and morality which until now have prescribed early universal marriage and continued childbearing throughout a woman's reproductive years.[83] Abortion has also not been a priority for those in charge of health and development programmes because of a lack of honesty, confidence and, until recently, information. Besides, decision-makers tend to be older males who lack empathy for the problem.

The equation of womanhood with motherhood arguably continues to underlie the 'invisibility of women' and their health needs outside of mothering.[84] This buttresses the definition of abortion as an illegal act and makes it less problematic to accept complications from abortion and even maternal mortality, since ill health becomes a 'natural' part of being a woman. It also leads to a lack of progress on a reproductive health agenda beyond that centred on child survival. Moreover, these problems are less likely to be addressed for the present because economic imperatives have driven fertility decline rather than a holistic change in behaviour that would include a broader understanding of women's health. Indeed, family planning service providers frequently lamented to the author how difficult it is to secure acceptance of family planning for health reasons. Larger changes in fertility preferences, family size and gender roles, as well as abortion policy, may have to await more substantial societal changes, particularly in regard to women's sense of autonomy. The act of abortion in a male-dominated society is not accepted until women reach a stage where they publicly recognize that they carry the burden of childbearing and choose to take command of their lives. While legislation facilitates these changes, they are not the result of laws or political activities; but without changes in legal and political practice, they will not occur.

A closely related reaction, rooted in the desire to re-establish control over women, would have it that 'abortion is undoubtedly a foreign imposition'.[85] Abortion is linked to 'loose women' or dismissed as a 'myth in nature'. Even prominent women have considered that abortion never occurred in the past.[86] Such claims are lent some credence, however spurious, by the shortage of studies on the topic. Nevertheless, it is clear that abortion was earlier practised across East Africa in accordance with 'the demands of the cultural institutions of a given ethnic group'.[87] Abortion occurred very discreetly and typically when taboos were broken rather than for newly apparent considerations, such as to complete one's education.

Such conflation is promoted by the clash between cultural trends, social changes, religious dogmas and political inertia. For example, there was no strong traditional argument against births out of wedlock, and women had more control of their own sexuality than in Christian cultures which placed virtue in female sexual restraint, especially premarital chastity, and distinguished between legitimate and illegitimate children.[88] This is another reason why with the recent expansion of schooling, adolescent sexuality and unwanted pregnancy have suddenly become major concerns amidst much confusion as to their management. Many teachers, parents, politicians and religious leaders, ignoring the implications of survey results, have held that contraceptives encourage adolescent promiscuity and abortion. The President himself seems caught in a tug of war between traditional influences and modernity. He has sought to reassure conservatives yet seems aware that family life education, however necessary, has proved 'too soft' and unsatisfactory by itself. The confusion compounds the problems associated with abortion, only some of which are beginning to be addressed under the rubrics of education and family planning.

Controversy over youth access to contraceptives and sex education has broadened and served, to some extent, as a euphemism for conflict over abortion. Whereas African and Christian pronatalist beliefs reinforced each other, colonial influences more strongly disturbed sexuality which continues to be affected by profound social changes, secular trends and Western media.[89] The most traumatic controversy between the missionary churches and their African converts occurred in the late 1920s and early 1930s over the rite of female circumcision, an issue recently revived by feminists and public health advocates.[90] The Christian stress on monogamous, indissoluble marriage was widely seen as an impossible demand, less consistent with the nature of human love or the aims of marriage than with 'the partisan adherence to a church with a set of unexplained laws and dogmas.'[91] It is plausible that sanctions against abortion will likewise come to be seen as legalistic ideals. Christian teaching on marriage, family life and sexuality is too weakly superimposed to replace the traditional customs and structures which have been destabilized. The resulting confusion is manifested in many ways, including the lack of consensus even on how to think about abortion, as well as the profound ambivalence over acknowledging young people's reproductive health concerns.

Other processes militate against major policy changes on abortion. These include the forces of inertia. Unsafe abortions are more prevalent in slums and back-door clinics than among the economically well-to-do. Clients and providers are linked in their interest to maintain confidentiality. There are many other pressing health problems competing for policy attention and limited resources. AIDS has now overtaken everybody and yet, as with sex education, it has proved difficult both to acknowledge the problem and to institute prevention programmes. At the same time, the law masks a strong religious conviction that abortion is unacceptable because of the biblical sanctity of life. Many ignore existing problems under a veil of moral and religious humility. In particular, Catholic opposition to abortion provides politicians a convenient lip-service for not raising their voice.

Kenya's elites show mixed and ambiguous attitudes towards abortion. Influential figures in public life have proved more politically conservative, elusive and less forthcoming and aggressive in pushing the issue than reformers would have liked. This is due to the sensitivities attached to abortion, the overall political environment, and because political conflicts in Kenya are often more personal than a matter of divergent policies and ideas. This lack of political development is another reason why it is difficult to construct a frame of reference and why many are unwilling to push matters further. Moreover, the state would want to be sure of support for any bold move to change the law on abortion. Likely partners, such as the medical profession or women's groups, are unwilling to stand up and argue with the facts at their disposal, and are divided in their opinions on the matter.

It is widely perceived that the authorities are aware that many abortions are being performed at considerable risk to health, but are insecure over the issue and are therefore not prepared to make major changes in abortion policy. Hence they tolerate and ignore the practice so long as it is quietly performed. This strategy, seemingly motivated by the desire not to 'rock the boat' and to minimize possible conflict, carries major public health disadvantages. Equally there is an unwillingness to consider the economic consequences of continuing with existing abortion policy. However, the costs of treating abortion-related complications and their long-term sequelae have yet to be thoroughly quantified in Kenya or anywhere else in Africa.

Church–state relations are still evolving and have been characterized by a wary cooperation that has become increasingly strained. Kenya is formally a secular state but, as in the USA, debate on the boundaries of separation remains unsettled. Both church and state have sought to avoid conflict, or at least reduce it to a minimum. Whereas Kenya's churches were reticent about becoming involved in political issues after independence, clergymen from the Catholic Church and some of the Protestant churches, particularly the Church of the Province of Kenya and the Presbyterian Church of East Africa, defended civil liberties more forcefully in the mid-1980s.[92] Both the regime and the *wanachi* ('the common man') came to see these churches as an unofficial opposition in the one-party state. Catholic leaders spoke out against the increasing identification of the ruling Kenya African National Union party (KANU) with the government, the legislative and judiciary branches; against abuses of power and corruption; and against the growing turmoil, tensions and injustices within Kenya. With the Pope commending his bishops for their strong defence of human rights,[93] the government has seemingly little to gain from a controversy with the Church over abortion, an issue which politicians do not consider a high priority.

Kenya is probably the only African state to have set up since independence a robust governance realm – where clear norms and procedures for regulating the relation between state and society provided a measure of accountability – only to dismantle it. Vice-President Moi assumed charge after Kenyatta's death in 1978 and refined his predecessor's autocratic grip. He has ruled in an increasingly personalized style, making abrupt policy and institutional changes.[94] Political life and administration remain patrimonial and clientelistic, with tight political control vested in the President and an extensive system of patronage firmly rooted in society. Government and bureaucracy were gradually fused into a single hierarchical power structure under the extended influence of KANU, as implied by the saying *'L'état, c'est Moi'*.[95] Accordingly, the political climate does not encourage free debate on most issues and policy initiatives are unlikely to be promoted without support at the highest level. In contrast to his support for family planning, President Moi has avoided talking about abortion and the problems of existing abortion policy. Few would venture to do so without such a cue. As one physician told the author, 'even a KMA chairman would feel constrained in giving information that may contradict the President'.

These are not the only systemic factors preventing abortion from assuming agenda status. A few years ago it seemed that abortion was working its way onto the national agenda, and whether it would be legal and under what circumstances would be resolved by Kenya's political process. Such a process did not halt because of a court decision, as in the USA.[96] Instead, customary Kenyan politics were disrupted by domestic and external communities who concluded that corruption, inefficiency and violence were endemic to Kenya and were excessively tolerated and encouraged by the President.[97] Although government critics and the relatively independent press continue to be intimidated, the reluctant acceptance of an autonomous sphere for the churches empowered civil society and the small activist opposition to push for change. By 1991 the severe economic decline had increased social hardships and triggered a political crisis. This emboldened the democracy movement calling for greater participation, accountability and material improvement. Following domestic and international pressure which included the partial suspension of Western aid, Moi's government grudgingly agreed to multiparty elections. The democratization process was checked, however, by a return to political authoritarianism and violence, a situation repeated ahead of the 1997 elections. The question of abortion has been postponed by all actors, including the state and the Catholic Church, as a side-effect of this internal instability and traumatic upheaval in Kenya's external relations. Not only has the abortion issue been upstaged by more fundamental political, economic and social questions, but in the present socio-political climate it would be a folly for any Kenyan leader to attempt to make it a national cause.

The overall political impasse has made for much haggling, a reluctance to take decisions, aloof and divided elites, and an apathetic and disaffected majority that feels helpless to bring up what it feels important. Aspiring reformers and those outside the 'system' find it difficult to lobby because public opinion is of little consequence and there have been so many personnel changes among the President's sycophantic supporters. It is hard to identify and work on influencing policymakers, not least over an issue still plagued by much ignorance among policymakers and ordinary people alike. As one frustrated gynaecologist told the author: 'If we mention the problems of unsafe abortion to the authorities, they still do nothing because this is the nature of things in Kenya.'

CONCLUSIONS

Abortion is emerging as an issue of policy concern in Kenya. Its practice is becoming more common, visible and recognized as a social reality, alongside much confusion over how it should best be understood and managed. Debate on abortion is still diffuse and intermittent, and the discourse poorly developed and not well focused; but debate has evolved from almost nothing within a short period of time, and the existence of many groups and external actors in Kenya is one of many reasons for thinking that there may be much conflict to come. This poses a challenge to the government in particular.

There are many reasons why, for now, abortion is not located higher on the agenda for action and which suggest that, for the foreseeable future, any changes in access to such services and the way in which abortion is considered are likely to be incremental. The reluctance to consider innovative reforms stems not from a conspiracy of silence as such, but primarily from widespread confusion as to how the question of abortion should be handled, as well as existing cultural, social and political sensitivities. These include public ideas concerning the roles of women and their marginalization, the gradual shrinking of the political arena, and the strained nature of church–state relations. The authorities find the current situation expedient and may not want to relax the law further, tolerating the provision of services so long as they are not openly advertised. The government, afraid of offending traditionalists and the churches, does not want to be seen as 'morally unsound'.

A number of external influences to this debate have been noted. To be accepted, however, the initiative for more innovative policy change has to come from within Kenyan society. Women's groups lack a powerful, coherent voice and a willingness to take the lead on this issue. Few physicians have done so, and medical bodies are not oriented as pressure groups. Like state and church, most groups wanting to bring about such change have been gripped by a pervasive fear of opening up a Pandora's box over abortion. As one potential reformer commented: 'Abortion is still a very sensitive subject and we do not want to burn our fingers overnight.' Various groups and individuals are working in a largely uncoordinated way towards a more liberal interpretation of the law, which is now less strictly enforced but may still cause problems for those working on its margins. Some of these policy entrepreneurs may seek to bring the abortion issue further into the public domain, most likely by focusing attention on the public health rationale for expanding existing services, with supporting grounds in the socio-economic dimension. Should discourse centre more strongly on morality, the Catholic Church's position will probably dominate and overshadow the secular debate.

The prospects for bold policy reform are unfavourable in the short term due to the ongoing political crisis and the weakness of communication channels with policymakers. While it is difficult to predict the future course of events, this chapter has identified a number of reasons why controversy seems likely to grow over abortion in Kenya, leading to greater demands for more substantial change in time to come and, quite possibly, a stronger counteraction to such proposals. In this way, the emergence of the abortion issue in Kenya may be a portent for other African countries.

3 Abortion in Mexico: Negotiating a Hidden Reality

In the early 1970s abortion was rarely discussed openly in Mexico. Since then, its intermittent appearance in public discourse has allowed for the gradual demystification of a once taboo subject. However, it is not yet possible to articulate all aspects of the issue and the question of abortion is mired in a state of negotiated reality where the problem is recognized but not addressed. While one might expect the state, the Catholic Church and those groups with an interest in this matter to become very active players in debate about abortion, it remains an issue where the risks seem greater than the gains to almost all of these parties. This condition induces them ordinarily to speak about abortion *sotto voce*.

As throughout Latin America, abortion in Mexico frequently occurs under unfavourable health conditions and in an environment that defines it as sinful and illegal. Laws on abortion in the region are, on paper if not in practice, among the most restrictive in the world.[1] Abortion is economically expensive for women who seek it and for the state which provides the services to treat complications that result from poorly performed procedures. Abortion is also a politically sensitive and difficult issue for both society and state. It is surprising therefore, that Mexican researchers and policymakers have examined the subject of abortion much less than might be surmised.

Mexico's relative stability, openness to social change, and intellectual tradition, have long been noted by other Latin American countries, underlining that 'the theme of Mexico leads to a reflection upon the fate of Latin America'.[2] In the early 1990s, the country featured strongly in the world's eyes as its young technocratic leaders negotiated the North American Free Trade Agreement (NAFTA), a common market with the USA and Canada, to deliver their country from underdevelopment. The country's size and growing international stature warrant close scrutiny. One could similarly almost expect that what happens in Mexico on abortion carries implications for the way abortion is regarded and treated elsewhere on the continent. Considerable energies have been periodically expended on changing laws and policies relating to abortion. However, it is unclear if there is a gradual tendency towards decriminalization, as certain trends suggest, or whether further change in that direction remains unlikely, given that groups hostile to the provision of abortion services have actively mobilized about the issue.

The most important of these actors is the Catholic Church. Mexico has the second largest national population of Catholics in the world and, despite the rapid spread of evangelical Protestantism in much of Latin America,[3] the continent remains crucial to the development of Catholicism and is its most populous region. Indeed, John Paul II made his first overseas trip as Pope to attend in Mexico the third meeting of the Latin American Episcopal Conference (CELAM III), the most powerful regional organization within the Catholic Church. In opening the conference, the Pope spoke of how families are threatened by 'campaigns advocating divorce, the use of contraceptives, and abortion, which destroy society'.[4] His characteristically forthright remarks came at a time when the Mexican church still had no legal status and the state had firmly committed itself to family planning. The Church and Church-backed groups have since become more assertive in their efforts to unseat family planning programmes, especially sex education, as well as in their denouncement of abortion. Abortion has been equated with contraception, as well as with the destruction of family values and structures. Although far fewer Mexicans practise their faith than are baptized, the Church's influence permeates social values and may increase in the public arena following the recent relaxation of anticlerical laws.

Mexico also has the second largest population in the region after Brazil. It has grown from less than 15 million in 1921 to 92 million in 1995 – more than in all of Central America and the Caribbean combined.[5] Birth rates, however, have fallen rapidly from 6.7 children per woman in 1970 to 3.0 in 1995, though there are marked geographic, residential and socio-economic differentials, and the annual population increment is over one million. The very youthful age structure suggests the need to extend contraceptive protection and accurate information so as to reduce the likelihood of unwanted pregnancy, especially among teenagers. Despite starting late in its efforts to control rapid population growth, Mexico was one of the first Latin American states to establish a national population council (CONAPO). The country developed into a major regional node in the worldwide operations of a number of family planning agencies. It also hosted the 1984 World Population Conference at which the USA announced its controversial decade-long 'Mexico City policy' that precluded foreign aid funds for any family planning agency that so much as mentioned abortion. Although no such agency engaged in abortion-related activities, the policy affected more sensitive components of family planning programmes in Mexico, such as contraceptive provision to youth, indirectly contributing to more unwanted pregnancies. Such adverse impacts explain why Mexicans have long said of their country in regard to its northern neighbour, with which it shares a long border and history: 'poor Mexico, so close to the USA, so far from God'. Relations between Mexico and the USA – like those between church and state – have warmed appreciably but remain complex. There continues to be widespread uneasiness about any partnership with a country that has figured in Mexican history more often as an adversary than as an ally.

Political power is concentrated in the executive office, following a tradition of strong rule that dates back to the Aztecs. This highly centralized level of policymaking is reflected in the design and implementation of the state's family planning programme and in the key role played in the nation's life by Mexico City, the fourth largest city in the world. The authoritarian, corporate structure severely limits political pluralism.[6] The Institutional Revolutionary Party (PRI), the world's longest governing party, has ruled since 1929 through patronage, electoral fraud, cooptation strategies and otherwise ensuring that opposition parties and groups are ineffectual. Its ideology has often changed in accordance with the dictates of the current president and circumstances. President Salinas (1988–94) presided over a modernization programme that renewed aggregate economic growth, patched up relations with the Church, and allowed a controlled, quasi-democratic discourse. His successor, Ernesto Zedillo, came to power just months after three unresolved events – an armed peasant revolt, the murder of the PRI's original presidential candidate, and major faction-fighting within the ruling party – shook the nation's institutions. Weeks later, a clumsy, forced currency devaluation brought on a severe economic crisis that further undermined confidence and deepened inequalities. In 1997 PRI lost its overall majority in the Chamber of Deputies and the mayoralty of Mexico City, and Mexico seemed to be slowly entering systemic change. Civil society has developed to the point where, as in much of Latin America, it must be considered alongside traditional political structures when analysing struggles taking place within the society and polity. The new social agents include feminist and anti-abortion groups. However, their avenues for expression remain restricted within a policymaking system that has always functioned beyond purview, as if behind a mask.[7]

This chapter assesses the existing abortion situation in Mexico and the surrounding policy context. It examines the roles played by different actors who have attempted to influence the course of abortion debate. It analyses why there has been so little substantive policy change on a subject long identified as a serious health and social problem inadequately resolved by existing policy measures. In interpreting why little has been done to come to terms with this hidden reality, I explain that the main impediments to such action lie in the continued marginalization of women, the inability of reform-minded groups to organize about this issue, the conservatism of political elites who are unlikely to risk confrontation with the Church hierarchy, and in the dominant modes of cultural and political praxis.

ACCESS TO ABORTION SERVICES

The Mexican legal system classifies abortion as a crime in most cases. Although there is no federal regulation, most states follow the example of the Federal District's 1931 penal code so that their criminal codes differ little from each other.[8] Abortion requires the approval of two physicians and is allowed only in the event of rape, incest, endangerment of the woman's life or imprudence (a term neither explained nor understood by the legal or medical profession, and which has no effect on access). In practice, cumbersome and bureaucratic practices and social and cultural barriers restrict access further. Interviews with lawyers, physicians, academics and social workers confirmed that some rape victims do not know that they can legally seek an abortion, let alone the procedure for obtaining one.

There are penalties for performing or procuring an illegal abortion, but their enforcement is almost unheard of.[9] The wording of the extenuating circumstances of liability (which reduces imprisonment if the woman is not of 'bad repute', manages to hide her pregnancy, and if it was the result of an illegitimate union) is common to most Latin American laws; the honour protected is essentially that of the husband the woman is considered to belong to, with her value depending on her virginity and fidelity. It would seem that the law preserves the mystification of motherhood and the myth of fidelity within marriage, while sanctions are not intended to be enforced if the abortion act is sufficiently masked.

The existing situation has several drawbacks. There are many unsafe abortions performed. The black market increases the economic and psychosocial costs of abortion for a woman. These should not be underestimated, because the decision to have an abortion is rendered more lonely and heavy by the socialization which makes women defer to men in general, yet holds them responsible for sexual relationships. Moreover, the law serves no useful purpose in reducing the incidence of abortion. It is exploitative and discriminates against poor women who cannot secure safe services that are available to the socio-economically advantaged.

As would follow, abortion is easier to obtain in a large city where there are more physicians, and women have a greater chance of securing anonymity. The most widely used method is dilatation and curettage; more dangerous methods include the 'sonda' (a rubber tube inserted into the uterus) and abortifacient herbs, a few of which may be quite effective. One particular plant (the 'cihuapahtli') acts as an abortifacient in strong doses; in smaller amounts, it is used as a contraceptive and to induce births.[10]

THE MEDICAL DEMOGRAPHY OF ABORTION

In Latin America, research interest in abortion waned once it was pointed out in the late 1960s and early 1970s that abortion was common and could be reduced through contraception.[11] It resurfaced two decades later, but the available pool of knowledge on abortion in Mexico, as for Latin America, is small, sketchy, and somewhat dated.[12] Abortion is greatly underreported owing to the illegality of the procedure, its social stigma and the failure to distinguish between spontaneous and induced abortions.[13]

In the late 1960s studies conducted on women covered by the health services of the Mexican Social Security Institute (IMSS, the largest health care provider) highlighted the widespread incidence of induced abortion and the high costs of attending to growing numbers of abortion complications in public hospitals. They also revealed that most women having abortions were multiparous house-wives who did so because they had an insufficient income or had already too many children. About 700,000 abortions occurred nationally.[14] This figure, while not rigorously computed, reflected informed opinion at a time when contraceptive use was still low in Mexico and abortion practice was already quite high in major ur-ban areas across Latin America. Although actual abortion rates remain unknown, they were undoubtedly significant as fertility de-clined rapidly in the 1970s and 1980s. Even after allowing for the rise in contraceptive prevalence that was occurring, induced abor-tion may have accounted for as much as one-quarter of deliberate fertility control over this period.[15]

A later estimate suggested that about 256,000 abortions were performed in Mexico during 1986, little more than twice the re-ported number of hospitalizations for abortion complications.[16] This implies that induced abortions averted a total of 138,000 births that year. Under this scenario, abortion rates peaked sometime earlier and their impact on fertility reduction has fallen. These estimates were not publicized for fear that they could give a false message of certainty and be used for political ends. The calculation is de-mographically elaborate, yet methodologically flawed. The index values and the age structure used to compute the induced abortion rates may not be representative. A higher incidence seems likely because contraceptive use and efficacy are still low, particularly in rural areas, despite the delivery and adoption of more effective contraceptive methods. Moreover, the proportion of abortions that require hospitalization is widely perceived to have fallen.

Another study suggested that 533,100 abortions occurred in Mexico in 1990. This implies an abortion rate of 23 per 1,000 women aged 15–49, slightly lower than that for the USA.[17] The calculation is based on the opinions of health workers and researchers from Mexico City and surrounding rural areas; and on a somewhat arbitrary in-flation factor of five abortions for every one treated in public hos-pitals. However, the same authors found in Bolivia, Colombia, Peru and Venezuela that hospitalizations from abortions performed else-where may be seven times higher than is officially reported.[18] Gynaecologists and physicians interviewed by the present author at several hospital sites in different Mexican cities believe they are seeing fewer cases of incomplete abortions than before; these patients are increasingly confined to the poor, lower middle-class and young, although many, if not most, are married with children. Along with other informed observers, obstetricians and gynaecologists also indicated that the incidence of abortion has probably not risen owing to increases in contraceptive use and, to some extent, in the cost of abortion.[19]

Most likely, there is substantial recourse to abortion in Mexico, but abortion rates are lower than the generally high levels thought to exist in much of Latin America. The decision to continue with an unwanted pregnancy may be easier in Mexico, where the ideal of motherhood is well ingrained and children are important to a woman's perception of integrity in a relationship. While abortion is increasingly identified by some as a problem among adolescents,[20] who may know of the existence of contraceptives but for various reasons are less likely to use them, it cannot be dismissed as a problem of reckless adolescents and single young women. Health care providers have often found that an adolescent who is negatively disposed towards her pregnancy or showing signs of rejection towards her child can be persuaded to feel otherwise.[21] Other research shows that most urban low- and lower-middle-income adolescents facing an out-of-wedlock pregnancy can adapt favourably to it given support from family and boyfriend.[22] Like non-use of effective contraception, this may reflect the limited alternatives and opportunities these adolescents see for their lives other than motherhood. Age at marriage and age at first child remain low, and women still receive a good deal of family support, even in Mexico City. A case-control study of adolescents (aged 15–19) hospitalized for incomplete abortion established that the absence of a mother from the pregnant adolescent's family background doubles the relative risk of an abortion, independent of the adolescent's education, the length of time she was in a union, and of the help she may have received in the process of seeking an abortion.[23]

There has always been much cross-border traffic by women seeking abortions, although this has been very poorly documented. Mexican clinicians ran thriving abortion practices that served many American women before the US Supreme Court legalized abortion,[24] after which thousands of Mexican women began travelling north for abortions. Employers in the northern border assembly plants (*maquiladoras*) often give pre-hiring pregnancy tests to avoid later paying maternity benefits and day-care expenses. Researchers, family planning and other health care providers in Ciudad Juárez confirmed to the author that the single young women who mostly work in these factories frequently resort to abortion to keep their jobs.

In the early 1990s IMSS extended the use of manual vacuum aspiration (MVA) to treat first trimester incomplete abortion patients and thereby reduce maternal mortality, morbidity and other costs. For 1987–89 at all IMSS facilities, maternal mortality ratios were estimated at 44.4 per 100,000 live births, one-fifth fewer than five years earlier. Abortion-related complications are reportedly the fifth leading cause of maternal death, down from 10 per cent of maternal deaths during 1984–86 to 7 per cent in 1988–90.[25] This decline may reflect improved treatment and fewer such admissions, perhaps due to better quality abortions being performed elsewhere; but these estimates may have always underestimated the true values and refer only to women seen at IMSS clinics, as most public and private hospitals do not report cases of incomplete abortion. Moreover, these estimates still imply that several hundred Mexican women may die each year from abortions performed elsewhere. Abortion-related deaths are often hidden as deaths due to infection, anaemia, renal failure or other causes, while patients with minor complications frequently do not request hospital treatment. There were 151 abortion-related maternal deaths registered in 1986; but a study by the Pan American Health Organization estimated a total of 5,138 maternal deaths in Mexico that year rather than 1,681 as officially reported. This gives a revised maternal mortality ratio of 200 (as opposed to 65) maternal deaths per 100,000 live births. A decade later, the World Health Organization put the number of maternal deaths at 2,700, yielding a maternal mortality ratio of 110 deaths per 100,000 live births, or a lifetime risk of maternal death of one in 220.[26]

THE PERPETUATION OF A PROBLEM

Abortion has become more problematic in Mexico not only due to the clash between groups seeking to determine the course of related public policy and the growing awareness of the public health risks stemming from the restrictive laws. The problem has been accentuated by the large unmet need for family planning, the neglect of women's reproductive health, changes in women's status and behaviour and, more slowly, in public attitudes toward women and sexuality. The exposure of various social myths surrounding abortion and sexuality, external influences and the growth in research interest and publicity have contributed as well. These factors underscore the pressing nature of existing problems, even if the question of how to manage abortion policy has only periodically come to the fore.

Although contraceptive prevalence has increased, there remains a large unmet need for family planning services which adds considerably to abortion practice. Among currently married women aged 15–49, the reported contraceptive prevalence increased from 30 per cent in 1976, to 53 per cent in 1987 and 67 per cent in 1995,[27] by when the contraceptive profile had begun to assume the 'mature' form typical for a developed country. In 1976, just under half (48 per cent) of currently married, non-pregnant and fecund women who wanted no more children were currently using contraception, as compared to an average of 57 per cent in Latin America and the Caribbean, and 87 per cent in 11 developed countries.[28] A decade later, there was still a high reliance on periodic abstinence and rhythm (8 per cent), with many barriers to more effective contraceptive use, especially in rural areas. The mean desired family size had fallen to 3.0, compared to an actual TFR of 3.8. These statistics imply that there are many unwanted pregnancies, or pregnancies that are not fully desired. One study estimated that 40 per cent of pregnancies in Mexico may be unwanted.[29]

Abortion was not publicly mentioned as a leading cause of maternal death until the government made use of the fact to justify its new population policy in 1974. While this opened up discussion about abortion, motherhood and sexuality, the government's intention was to generate support for the new family planning programme rather than to soften up the ground for reforming abortion policy. Although the state has since rhetorically stressed women's equality and integrated family planning services with those of maternal and child health (MCH), women in general continue to be disadvantaged in terms of health and unwanted fertility.

Significant changes have occurred over the past two decades in the status of women and in women's sexuality. Younger, urban women are now better educated, more likely to be salaried, and less dependent on their parents. This makes them better able to formulate more diverse goals and to question their traditionally engendered roles, as well as related public policy. This does not mean that such changes are fully accepted. In many quarters there is still a disapproval of women having sexual relations for pleasure rather than for procreation, and adolescent sexuality outside of marriage continues to be denied in a society where over one-fifth of the population is between 10 and 19 years of age. A number of socio-cultural pressures continue to push Mexican youth towards early marriages and early pregnancies. Many young people remain poorly informed on contraception and reproduction, contributing to wide-spread unprotected sex and unintended pregnancy. Among young adults (aged 15–24) in Mexico City who had completed secondary education by 1985, only 40 per cent of women and 30 per cent of men could identify the most fertile period during the woman's menstrual cycle, yet rhythm was the most commonly used method among the sexually active.[30] The situation has probably improved since, but NGOs struggle to fill the gaps created by obstacles to implementing and expanding family planning policies.

Mexican elites follow closely what happens in the USA, although deep sensitivities to foreign intervention prevent this from being acknowledged. It would be wrong, however, to overstate these in-fluences; the legalization of abortion in the USA in 1973 did not affect legal developments in Mexico where major policy changes are unthinkable without a decision taken at the very top of the political system. Nevertheless, Mexican officials are keenly aware that US presidents moved vigorously in the 1980s to restrict access to abortion. This may account for some of their own reluctance to consider abortion-related problems and has made it extremely difficult for NGOs to address the issue. The influences of the Catholic Church's transnational linkages are discussed later.

Mexico has been affected by the growing international aware-ness that abortion is a major health problem for women. By the early 1990s this became evident in the activities of several small players in the abortion debate. IPAS, a US-based NGO, had helped introduce MVA equipment to improve the management of incom-plete abortion. Both the Population Council and the Ford Founda-tion sponsored reproductive health programmes stressing research on abortion. In its own small way, this work seems to have refo-cused attention on the issue, brought together individuals working in separate institutions, and added to the discussion of public health and women's choices.[31]

Recent opinion polls indicate greater public acceptance of abor-tion than had been assumed, though no consensus exists. A 1991 Gallup poll conducted in the three largest cities (Mexico City, Guadalajara and Monterrey) found that 43 per cent of people be-lieve that the decision to have an abortion belongs to the woman alone; 48 per cent think that women need not take into account the church's opinion when deciding about such a procedure; and 77 per cent consider that legalizing abortion could prevent the deaths of many women. However, only 38 per cent of people support the idea that health care institutions should provide abortion services. Those of age 21 to 35 and residents of Mexico City hold the most liberal attitudes, but there is little differentiation by sex and socio-economic status.[32] This widely publicized survey exposed various social and cultural myths about abortion. These are proving very hard to dispel, like other mores about appropriate and standard sexual behavior. Research findings may help move the issue of abortion on to the public platform, but they have not swayed public opinion, which to date has exerted little direct influence on Mexican policymakers.

THE COURSE OF THE ABORTION DEBATE

We can distinguish five phases in the course of debate on abortion since the mid-1970s.[33] While the publication of several research papers stimulated some professional debate on the problem,[34] abortion first moved onto the agenda through the efforts of the emerging feminist movement and as a result of the discussion surrounding the state's introduction of a new population policy. The government recognized the right to family planning and set up a strong family planning programme, justified in part through the need to reduce the high number of abortions. A government-commissioned study favoured legalizing abortion,[35] but submitted its testimony just before a presidential succession when little was likely to be accomplished. The suggestions were not followed and the 'expert dialogue' soon ended.

A new phase in the debate began when left-wing parties were legalized at the end of the decade. The new President distanced himself from the abortion issue, which soon became radicalized as the focus of an alliance between feminists and communists. They proposed a law on 'voluntary motherhood' (*maternidad voluntaria*), referring to a woman's right to choose to have children.[36] It set out to legalize abortion within the first trimester, as had become law in the USA six years earlier, to regulate its practice within the Sanitary Code and to promote sex education and family planning. However, differences deepened among the sponsors of the measure and the draft legislation was frozen in committee and never publicly discussed by government circles.[37] The feminist movement, the strongest backer of abortion rights, virtually collapsed as a result of its unsuccessful cooperation with the much vilified Communist Party. The Church, buoyed by the visit of the Pope in 1979, voiced its objections more publicly than when the state instituted a national family planning programme. A church-linked organization, Pro-Vida ('Pro-Life'), was formed to forestall legalization of abortion and set out to assume a role as a guardian of the nation's moral conscience. With Church assistance it mobilized people to march in the streets, a form of protest feared by Mexican governments, especially since the 1968 Tlatelolco massacre when federal troops shot scores of students in Mexico City.

The third development can be characterized as a 'dialogue of the deaf'. In the course of the 1982 presidential campaign, the incoming President Miguel de la Madrid proposed to decriminalize abortion. He referred to abortion as an 'outstanding' issue that should be 'considered dispassionately ... with a view to giving [women] truly free choices and protecting their health', and added that a referendum on the matter 'must be conducted in due course'.[38] However, few spoke out in favour of the idea which was dropped once it encountered opposition from the National Action Party (PAN), Pro-Vida and the Church. The deep economic crisis dominated the political scene and created political opportunities best exploited by conservative groups, with whom the new government augmented its links.

A fourth and very different debate took place after police raided an abortion clinic in Mexico City over Holy Week 1989. Although the police had blackmailed service providers and clients before, this time several of the arrested women publicly denounced the police action and expressed their support for legalized abortion services; so did over 700 elite women who signed a widely publicized declaration which showed that feminists and non-feminists could cross ideological, party and class lines over this issue.[39] This triggered another debate on abortion and legal inequities that, unlike before, took place in the public sphere and was not consciously manufactured by the government. Those opposed to such a policy shift were divided. Some PAN deputies abstained out of principle, being against the arbitrary use of force, whereas the bishops and Pro-Vida were now cast in a radical light for having supported the raids. At the same time, the Attorney General's Office prepared a revised draft of the Penal Code, whose antecedents lay in a 1983 draft that would have allowed abortion on grounds of poverty.[40] The new proposal again failed to reach Congress, but was undoubtedly discussed at the governmental level. It would have kept abortion criminal but contained loopholes allowing a judge not to jail a woman who had carried it out, thereby bringing the law closer in line with existing practice.[41]

A fifth period concerns the huge controversy that flared up when it was announced in December 1990 that the Chiapas state legislature, dominated by the long-ruling PRI, had revised its abortion law two months earlier. Legislators said they acted on behalf of thousands of women suffering injury, infertility or death from clandestine unhealthy abortions. The state attorney repeated to the author that 200,000 abortions occurred each year in Chiapas,[42] an implausibly high number first publicized by the state governor. The revised law stated that abortion would not be punished during the first 90 days of gestation if the pregnancy resulted from rape, placed the woman at risk of death or showed evidence of foetal defects; when the abortion was carried out for reasons of family planning if the couple had agreed to the procedure, or in the case of a single woman, if she had obtained medical consent.[43] The Catholic Church and Church-linked organizations reacted swiftly and sharply. Although the incident re-galvanized feminist voices in support of abortion rights, the central government would not have wanted to risk new obstacles in the way of mending church–state relations. Within two weeks the Chiapas state legislature had suspended the process. Proponents and opponents of reform then besieged the National Human Rights Commission, a federal ombudsman that ultimately reports to the president and which avoided ruling on whether the revision violated human rights.

Many observers consider the move to have been a kite flown by President Salinas, a normally very decisive man. Mexico's southernmost and poorest state offered a setting where dispute could be contained because of its distance from the capital, relatively low profile within national life, lack of a Catholic tradition, high incidence of abortion-related illness, and the specific nature of church–state relations and of internal church relations within Chiapas itself. The State Governor had long been at odds with the well-known Catholic Bishop of San Cristóbal de las Casas, a strong supporter of the rights of indigenous peoples and considered by the Church's more conservative hierarchy as a spokesperson for Mexico's liberation theologians. The state may have wanted to promote a progressive image to divert attention from its administrative failures within Chiapas. It may have also thought the Church hierarchy would consider its developing dialogue with the Salinas administration threatened by the bishop, an eloquent opponent of the NAFTA trade agreement. The Governor's action may have been further prompted by an eventful CONAPO meeting one month earlier, at which the President reminded his governors that family planning targets were to be met and conspicuously departed when the recipient of a demographic prize criticized the lack of investment in key social sectors, particularly health and education.[44]

The importance of the Chiapas episode may lie in its legacy. The state legislature had passed Mexico's most liberal abortion statute which, when challenged, was not repealed but put on hold. For the first time public discussion of abortion was not confined to specific groups or forums. The extensive media comment included a widely viewed, six-hour-long television debate involving prominent figures holding differing views about abortion, a subject still partly taboo until then.[45] In 1993 abortion was again discussed in political circles as the focus of special sessions of the Chamber of Deputies' Health Commission, but all the major presidential candidates in the 1994 election avoided the issue.

THE SOCIAL CONSTRUCTION OF ABORTION

Debate on abortion is poorly informed by basic facts. An analysis of newspaper coverage over the period 1974 to 1982 revealed major inconsistencies in the numbers and rates cited for abortion incidence and cause-related mortality, but reasonable congruency in the reported profile characteristics of abortion patients.[46] Estimates of the incidence of abortion ranged from 50,000 to 6 million, those of maternal deaths varied from 5,000 to 400,000, and 39 per cent of the figures cited did not mention their sources. The results underscore the failure of the health and research communities to address these matters further.

Although articles favouring legalizing abortion are more likely to use statistics to justify their argument, the value of data is now being recognized by Pro-Vida. Its Women's Aid Center in Mexico City has started to collect basic statistics on women who come for pregnancy counselling, sometimes thinking they will obtain an abortion. Such women are said to be mostly single and young. They are twice as likely to seek abortion on social as compared to economic grounds, and nine times more than for health reasons.[47] It remains to be seen whether such data can discredit alternative discourses that use statistics. Research two decades ago identified women who had abortions as mostly married with children, contradicting prevailing social myths surrounding abortion. It also pressed recognition of abortion as a public health issue. Arguably, such a case for reviewing abortion policy has not been presented strongly. However, public health concerns are not accorded high priority and tend to enter political discourse only rhetorically. As the case of AIDS illustrates, strong latent prejudices about behavioural practices have often reduced public health campaigns to generalities, platitudes or fear tactics, particularly where issues touch on the sexual sphere.

Many observers feel that society is now more open to discussing abortion. However, public debate has tended to be episodic and marked by many polemical arguments, underscoring a profound 'clash' of views. The substance and the language of the abortion debate have changed little over time. Interest in abortion is often not shown directly even though the issue has been politicized to some extent. This stems from the restrictions imposed on civil society; the primordial association of abortion with blood and the 'feminine', and its inelegance for a heavily male-dominated culture; the divisive and difficult nature of the issue; and the preference of many Mexicans for more indirect ways of expression and negotiation rather than open conflict. That the subjective is a key element in Mexican political praxis helps explain why the question of abortion has been raised only obliquely by several administrations. It is also the reason why a number of reform advocates – such as the Reproductive Rights Information Group, GIRE, founded in 1992 – seek to negotiate the decriminalization of abortion, rather than outspokenly demand the liberalization of abortion *per se*. In the process, they are trying to make abortion the concern of society, not just of feminists, and to communicate an alternative position by stressing the language of choice and greater tolerance.[48]

There is no clear framework for thinking about abortion, reflecting the lack of societal consensus and the multiplicity of views and opinions that have been exchanged. Some public officials think of abortion as a public health problem or relate it to the issue of population growth, but the Chiapas controversy showed that there is considerable resistance – from feminists and the Church alike –

to defining abortion as a demographic issue. Beyond Mexico City and outside of intellectual circles, few think of abortion as an aspect of freedom and rights, even if there is a greater willingness to talk about abortion and women's choices. Groups seeking to remove restrictions on abortion services have based their arguments on public health and social justice considerations, as well as a woman's right to control her own body. However, earlier calls for the right to voluntary motherhood changed neither the language nor the terms of debate. Recent discourse on reproductive rights has added to discussion about abortion, but groups seeking to liberalize abortion services are finding it difficult to sustain debate and extend it to such issues as sexuality and education.

The Catholic Church, which has acted as an umbrella for conservative opposition to abortion, has attempted to keep debate focused instead on the ontological status of the foetus. Church rhetoric suggests that life begins at the moment of conception and that abortion kills an innocent person. Its teaching presupposes that a woman's love and life are self-sacrificial before the foetus. To this, the Church adds that abortion should not be legalized because nearly all Mexicans are (baptized) Catholic and, perforce, follow and agree with this teaching. The view that abortion is a sin remains an important defining construct, underlining widespread compliance with a social Catholicism.

Several other interconnected socio-cultural elements underpin considerations of abortion. These include public ideas about gender roles, motherhood and sexuality. As in the USA, a strong undercurrent to this debate is the concern with women's roles and lives. In particular, abortion contradicts the idealization of motherhood that lies at the core of women's identity. In 1988 at least two out of every five women (45 per cent) considered that the most important goal in their lives was 'to have children'.[49] The somewhat dated stereotypes of 'machismo' and of the passive dependent woman are not particularly useful in understanding this ideal; yet in spite of expanded opportunities and goals, a woman's role is still popularly conceived as mother and homemaker, and double standards of sexual morality remain common. This makes it easier for conservative groups to confront feminist calls for 'voluntary motherhood' and reproductive rights, since many people find it threatening to the social and cultural order.

This order is symbolized by the evocative Catholic symbols of motherhood and suffering, particularly in Marian imagery and devotion. At the outset of his papacy, John Paul II visited the Basílica of Guadalupe, the patroness of Mexico and symbol of national pride, and compared her to the Black Madonna of Częstochowa, who holds a similar niche in Polish nationalism and culture.[50] Women generally continue to be held responsible for the contraceptive ignorance and failure that lead to unwanted pregnancy, and, despite the mystification of motherhood, the government does not support the needs of many mothers. The political culture continues to privilege the rights of the group over the individual, making it difficult to advance the limited autonomy and minority status of women.

The state has not formed its own discourse on abortion, in contrast to its concern about population growth and for family planning which, it asserts, reduces abortion. The state has mediated between the actors engaged in the dispute and set the parameters of the debate. However, the state's recent inability to defuse promptly conflicts over police raids on abortion clinics and over legal initiatives shows its control is far from total. Successive governments have tested the waters for reform and, on occasion, declared that abortion is a public health issue, but they have refused to take sides publicly in the dispute, or to exert a commanding say, except in so far as to postpone possible reforms repeatedly.

The next sections examine the role played by the key non-governmental actors in the abortion debate. Greatest attention is given to the Catholic Church in the light of its deep roots in Mexican culture, its strong organizational base throughout the country, its longstanding interest in this issue, and its new assertiveness.

THE MEXICAN CATHOLIC CHURCH AND THE ABORTION QUESTION

Church–state relations

The role played by the Catholic Church in influencing abortion policy, discourse and trends cannot be understood outside the historical context of church–state relations. The separation of church and state was established by the 'Reforma' of the late 1850s and reinforced by the 1917 revolutionary constitution.[51] Church–state relations have been marked by conflict over education, the Church's civil status and role in Mexican life, and the extent of the state's authority. Until the Church regained full legal status and the state restored diplomatic ties with the Vatican in 1992, they have been governed by a *modus vivendi* whereby the state did not enforce anti-clerical laws while the Church stayed clear of the political forum and was expected to help keep social order. At the same time the clergy maintained influence by developing a network of lay organizations, such as the National Parents' Union, and implicitly supporting PAN, the voice of national conservatism which has favoured Church activism. Perhaps more importantly, it has played a major and under-examined role in educating Mexican elites through private church schools and colleges.[52] The social values associated with the Catholic tradition remain embedded, if not necessarily thriving, within the dominant culture. This is why the Church can still count on many devout followers, in spite of growing secularization.

In the 1960s the turmoil of the Second Vatican Council in Rome and the second conference of Latin American bishops (CELAM II) in Medellín, Colombia, found only a muted echo among Mexico's hierarchy.[53] It remained deeply conservative and established increasingly conciliatory relations with successive governments in the 1970s. The bishops did not openly confront the state's adoption of an anti-natalist population policy,[54] because the Church's constitutionally disadvantaged status precluded them from publicly pronouncing on social issues. The Mexican Episcopal Conference assumed a greater public role in the 1980s due to the political bankruptcy, economic mismanagement and unpopularity of PRI, as well as the electoral gains made by PAN. It was also spurred by the impact of a new Pope who strongly advocated respect for human rights, and the perception that the state's new technocratic leaders would not retaliate against the Church. The relaxation of state-imposed restrictions on church activities has enabled the clergy to mobilize considerable support at the local and national level when deemed important, as during the Chiapas controversy.

The Church resurfaced as a political power through negotiating with President Salinas. He saw that abandoning official anti-clericalism could help him consolidate his power following a disputed election and broaden his support base to carry out reforms.[55] It is unclear what, in addition to its legal rights, the Church may have asked for in exchange for its support; one can only speculate if the issue of abortion was a bargaining point. The Church then called AIDS education and family planning programmes 'abuses of power'[56] and

pressured the government AIDS council (CONASIDA) to abandon a campaign to promote condom use. Family planning leaders
expressed to the author a great deal of concern that their programmes
have since become politically neglected and inadequately protected
from attacks by increasingly powerful conservative groups. In late
1991 the National Parents' Union criticized proposals to update
sex education classes, leading the Ministry of Education to drop
the planned revisions. Six months later, conservative groups succeeded for the first time ever in forcing the state to suspend a
family planning programme. A series of charges were mounted against
MEXFAM (the national IPPF affiliate), public sector family planning programmes and AIDS-prevention efforts in the ordinarily quiet
state of San Luis Potosí. The local Pro-Vida chapter, set up just
months earlier, glued together a coalition of civic and Catholic-
based groups that prevailed on the reluctant governor to select
MEXFAM as a sacrificial lamb and suspend its activities within
the state. The governor, piously compared to Pontius Pilate for
having 'washed his hands' of the issue, called his accusers 'false
redeemers' in turn.[57]

Church-based opposition to abortion

In 1980 the government invited the Church to address the Commission on Health and Welfare then considering possible changes
in the abortion law. The invitation was cancelled following bitter
objections from individuals and groups, although the hierarchy insisted its voice should be heard on the grounds that it represents
90 per cent of the population and that abortion is a moral rather
than a political question.[58] The protests highlighted the continued
sensitivities surrounding church–state relations and clergy opinion
over issues neither strictly moral nor religious. Mexican bishops
and Pro-Vida condemned abortion and contraception when the idea
of legalizing abortion was mooted in 1982–83 and at the time of
the 1984 World Population Conference. The bishops disclosed a
message sent by the Pope to the conference Secretary-General, which
asserted that rich countries were unjustly conditioning aid to poor
countries on the acceptance of 'contraception, sterilization and
abortion programs that violated individual freedoms and contributed to an anti-life mentality'.[59] The Mexican government adopted
a low-key stance at the next such decennial conference held in Cairo,
when Church officials pressed it to oppose forcefully the liberal

consideration of abortion policy proposed in the preparatory conference document.[60]

The Church hierarchy and other conservative sectors more sharply rebuked the earlier domestic initiative to legalize abortion in Chiapas. Twenty local deputies who voted in favour of the reforms were excommunicated and compared to the 'army of Saddam Hussein which killed babies they found in incubators during the invasion of Kuwait'.[61] The National Action Party and San Cristóbal's outspoken bishop accused PRI of caving in to pressure from the International Monetary Fund and the World Bank to control Mexico's population growth in return for an increase in the nation's credit line against its huge foreign debt. The Papal Nuncio – who played a key role in renegotiating church–state relations and has publicly denounced abortion on several occasions since his appointment in 1990 – called upon President Salinas to override the state action. Pro-Vida continued to rally opposition to the measure long after it was suspended, deriving strength from the momentum held by anti-abortion groups in the USA at the time. It organized a march to the palace of the President and petitioned him to reverse the initiative; despite deferring any judgment on the matter, his office promptly published a decree that reflected the spirit of the 1989 UN Convention on the Rights of the Child.[62] Pro-Vida demanded a constitutional amendment ensuring the right to life from the moment of conception, reflecting similar guarantees instituted in the neighbouring Central American states of Guatemala and Honduras, as well as Ecuador. One prominent bishop stated: 'A true democracy has to defend the rights of the people and the first right of all people is the right to life. The right to life from the womb should be elevated to a constitutional level.'[63]

The Episcopal Commission for the Family promotes Church teaching on the family. Its board includes representatives of various Catholic groups and religious orders who vigorously oppose abortion under any circumstances. The commission's President – since appointed as Archbishop of Mexico City, the largest diocese in the world – explained to the author that it seeks to stop publications and media messages 'dealing with AIDS, sex education, non-natural methods of family planning, as promoted by NGOs and sometimes by the government, and which are part of the worldwide plan to undermine such [Catholic] values'.[64] Through its pastoral letters, the Church has called for the protection of all human life and has rallied against abortion and 'artificial contraception', contrasting 'family planning' to 'responsible parenthood'.[65]

It is by no means certain if Mexican Catholics are listening closely to these injunctions.[66] Pro-Vida representatives admitted privately to the author that even some priests are unsure what Pro-Vida stands for. Most Catholics neither attend church regularly nor practise their faith rigidly. As in Poland, some Catholic women have more qualms about using contraception than resorting to abortion, owing to a peculiar interpretation of Catholic rationalism. A woman confessing to an abortion has only to request a pardon once and she is forgiven, whereas she would be repeatedly sinning if she used contraception.[67] The Church has not promoted natural family planning methods as actively as in Kenya or Poland, although it cooperates with closely linked groups such as 'Fame' (the youth arm of the Legionaries of Christ, a religious order) and the Billings National Center.[68] Mindful of its perceived insensitivity to the plight of women with crisis pregnancies, in contrast to its professed love for the unborn and readiness to condemn abortion, Pro-Vida set up ten Women's Aid Centers between 1989 and 1992 which attended to some 4,000 women.[69]

Since its foundation in 1978, when pro-life groups began to flourish in the USA, Pro-Vida has frequently assailed family planning programmes and mobilized against initiatives deemed antithetical to 'family values'. By 1993 its formal structure extended to nearly all 31 states beyond the capital. The group's leaders told the author they do not see the US pro-life movement as a model because certain behaviours, such as the militant grassroots activism of Operation Rescue, are illegal in Mexico. However, Pro-Vida publicly exposes physicians and clinics said to be carrying out abortions. One former director of Mexico's largest family planning programme described Pro-Vida to the author as 'the civil armed force of the Catholic Church'.[70] It is by far the most energetic of anti-abortion groups. Two others with a national structure are the National Parents' Union, which focuses on youth education, and 'Ancifem' (the National Civic Association of Women), created in 1984 to combat perceived feminist threats to traditional female roles. Although now less vigorous as an organization, Ancifem has become closely tied to the National Action Party and has a solidly middle-class female membership. 'Vida Humana' is a Mexico-City-based group that used to cooperate closely with Human Life International (from the USA). It is closely linked with the Church and published its first newsletter in 1991.

According to the Vatican, over two million people are involved in the large lay movements which account for much of the Church's vitality.[71] These include arch-conservative orders such as the Legionaries of Christ and Opus Dei, both of which help Pro-Vida.[72] Opus Dei is an influential part of the body politic across Latin America. It directs a number of educational institutions in Mexico, where it has penetrated universities and seminaries, and made its presence felt in the upper levels of public administration. Members of Opus Dei strongly oppose abortion which they consider to be just one step away from contraception. The Knights of Columbus, a fraternal Catholic group with significant resources, also assists Pro-Vida.

External linkages

The Vatican views Mexico as pivotal to the diffusion of orthodox belief in Latin America. By 1998 John Paul II had visited Mexico three times, his first trip being a triumphant tour similar to that he was about to make to his native Poland. Millions greeted him across the republic, at once demonstrating the Church's latent power and the contempt in which the constitution and public authority were held. The Pontiff likened the Mexican and Polish churches, which both had to deal with authoritarian states. He also made clear his support for human rights and criticized the use of contraceptives and abortion. Emboldened by his example, the Mexican hierarchy spoke out more on social issues, including *maternidad voluntaria*, and increasingly associated itself with demands for electoral democracy. About 30 million people saw the Pope during his second visit in 1990 that began another round of trips to the countries of Latin America and the Caribbean. The Pope again railed against contraception and abortion. His visit also implied tacit support for the new government and hastened the pace of church–state reforms. John Paul II paid a brief third visit in 1993 to address Amerindian groups in Mexico's southeast, who are much courted by evangelical Protestants, and then attended the World Youth Day festival in the USA where he castigated abortion and contraception once more.

The Pope's remarks on birth control underscore the degree to which the Vatican, the Mexican hierarchy and Pro-Vida consider Mexico to be a strategic point in the worldwide struggle over abortion. Prominent churchmen and anti-abortion activists insist the government is under strong international pressures to reduce demographic growth by all means, including abortion, and point out that Mexico is a regional node for family planning organizations working in Latin America. They repeatedly stated to the author that legalization of abortion would open the door to similar moves within the region.

Pro-Vida held national congresses, meetings of its youth wing and two international conferences in the late 1980s attended by leading figures from the Mexican church and the US anti-abortion movement.[73] Pro-Vida has proved adept at initiating and developing contacts. These are very strong and direct with senior Mexican bishops and the Vatican, which is aware that Pro-Vida could serve as a regional model. In a written message, the Pope extolled participants to its first international congress to 'make society see the importance of defending life from the moment of conception up to death'.[74] At the Vatican's request, Pro-Vida and the Episcopal Commission for the Family jointly organized the first Latin American regional pro-life conference in Monterrey in 1992. Pro-life representatives from 22 Latin American countries, Spain, Italy, and France attended the meeting, as did cardinals from Mexico, Latin America and the Vatican. They included Colombian Cardinal Alfonzo López Trujillo, the Secretary of the Pontifical Council for the Family and past president of CELAM who, in that capacity, was instrumental in suppressing the continent's liberation theology movement with the help of Opus Dei.[75] Conference participants judged the meeting favourably for its publicity, the networking and exchange of information it allowed, and the prospect of increased cooperation between national churches, CELAM and church-linked organizations.

The Pope, who sent messages of support to all three international Pro-Vida congresses, received a delegation from Pro-Vida one month later in Rome. He then summoned all Latin American bishops in charge of their national family life commissions.[76] Mexican links with the Vatican's vast information network remain strong despite the 1993 slaying of the Cardinal of Guadalajara, a member of the Pontifical Council for the Family.[77] In 1996 this council convened in Mexico City a meeting attended by politicians, legislators and leaders of anti-abortion groups from every American country.[78] Contacts between Mexican and US church sources are said to be good. The Knights of Columbus regularly invite Mexican bishops to their US national conferences, where abortion has been discussed alongside genetics, family values and structures. Pro-Vida personnel acknowledge the help given by some US Catholics in setting up their first Women's Aid Center, and the written and audio-visual materials sent by the US-based group Human Life International. They now envisage playing a similar supportive role to Central and Latin American groups who share their agenda.

Dissenting Catholicism

Several Catholic groups have recently attempted to open up debate about their Church's teaching on women, sexuality and reproductive health, including abortion. Catholics for a Free Choice is a small but active group that publishes a quarterly opinion journal on these matters, along the lines of its US parent organization. It has started to receive attention from the Mexican press and has earned the wrath of the institutional Church.[79] The alternative strand of Catholic thought it represents is not well known in Mexico, and it possesses almost no resources compared to the Church hierarchy. Other groups calling for a greater dialogue within the Church command an even smaller public presence and refrain from directly questioning official teaching on abortion. Their existence, however, shows that a plurality of opinions exists within the Church, despite initial appearances to the contrary.

The ability of non-governmental actors to push for a more liberal abortion policy is hindered by existing abortion laws, concerns about church-based opposition, and the limits on associational life set by the state. However, such groups do have spaces in which to operate, as examined below.

REFORMIST VOICES IN THE ABORTION DEBATE

The feminist challenge for abortion rights

Feminists have been by far the most vocal advocates of legalizing abortion. Their struggle began in earnest in the 1970s. It was aided by awareness of the growth of the feminist movement in the USA and Western Europe, the government's new rhetorical commitment to gender equality that marked its reversal on population policy, and the staging of the 1975 UN Conference on Women in Mexico City. However, the loose-knit feminist coalition has been beset by deep longstanding internal divisions, strategic errors, and organizational problems.[80]

Feminist activism peaked in the late 1970s, when demands for the legalization of abortion figured prominently in the formation of various action groups, notably the Coalition of Feminist Women, and in the leading feminist journal, *Fem*. Differences developed over whether to push for decriminalization alone or abortion on demand; what time limit to seek under which an abortion should be permitted without restriction (in the late 1970s many feminists wanted it to be as unrealistically long as the full nine months of gestation); and how best to pursue such claims. The purist convictions held by feminist leaders, and their understandable fears of being coopted and neutralized by the PRI, made it even more difficult to succeed in a *de facto* one-party system. The cooperation with the communist parliamentary faction in 1979 has stigmatized feminists to this day. The Chiapas controversy showed they still cannot rely on the political left for support and have not managed to exploit their opportunities. The feminist movement remains splintered and elitist in a class-ridden society,[81] failing to absorb young people and to speak meaningfully to the mass of women it claims to represent. Their concerns are more often rooted in basic economic needs and reflected in the demands of many other women's activists which, for the most part, are not integrated into an understanding of gender oppression. Feminist leaders have also failed to negotiate closer ties with the Ministry of Health.

In an attempt to be more effective and to avoid speaking as separate cliques talking among themselves, several women's rights activists formed the group GIRE about the same time that the state modified the legal status of religious institutions. GIRE seeks to advance a reproductive rights agenda that stresses the public health and social justice reasons for revising abortion policy. As part of its aims to promote action-oriented research and disseminate information, GIRE has jointly sponsored with Gallup, the US-based polling organization, several well-publicized surveys of attitudes on abortion in Mexico. GIRE has developed links with several family planning agencies as well as activist and educationally oriented groups such as Catholics for a Free Choice, and lobbied deputies and senators.[82] By 1996, four years after its foundation, GIRE employed 16 staff members and commanded good contacts with journalists who increasingly reported its opinions in juxtaposition to those of the Church. Whether GIRE can build on its initial successes remains to be seen.

Physicians and family planning agencies

In Mexico, as throughout Latin America, physicians have long been aware of the large numbers of women hospitalized for abortion-related complications, but once they provided a health-based justification for establishing family planning primarily in terms of reducing abortion, they refrained from further say in how abortion should be handled.[83] Mexican physicians have been remarkably mute throughout the course of the abortion debate. Although they feel they can legitimately decide on matters of women's health and fertility, many male professionals in dominant positions do not ascribe high priority to abortion problems. Even if they did, Mexican physicians do not collectively command strong influence. As in Poland and Kenya, interviews with physicians revealed a resistance on the part of health care providers to giving proper care. This may stem from personal convictions about appropriate reproductive conduct and is manifested in different ways; even the quality of hospital registration forms differs between those women admitted for an incomplete abortion and those admitted for a caesarean section or a normal delivery, underlining that abortion patients are usually treated as second-class patients.

Some physicians clearly do not accept the implications of the statistics collected on abortion-related morbidity and mortality; many are as ambivalent about abortion as the rest of society. A good portion of gynaecologists and other physicians maintain silence on the subject because they illegally profit from it; others stay quiet for fear of being stigmatized with doing so. The medical profession has never attempted to influence abortion policy and is unlikely to do so unless it becomes more powerful and policymakers are perceived as more receptive to the issue. Physicians are largely apolitical, neither working individually nor through their professional organizations to effect change. The National Academy of Medicine and the Mexican Federation of Gynecological and Obstetrical Associations have never issued a statement on abortion.[84]

Family planning agencies have not played a more pro-active role in abortion care for various political (domestic and international), cultural and social reasons. The attack on MEXFAM (the Mexican Foundation for Family Planning) has underscored the hazards of working in what is a difficult political environment. Even if they are willing to consider the issue of abortion, family planning agencies for the most part exhibit a 'cultural bias' against involvement in abortion-related work. Their focus is on the technical aspects of contraceptive service delivery, not on the termination of an existing pregnancy. All are worried about engaging in public debate about abortion. The US 'Mexico City policy' of the 1980s further slowed attempts to tailor contraceptive services to the needs of post-abortion patients.[85]

Researchers and journalists

Academics and other researchers have tended to overlook the question of abortion. There are several reasons for this. The state has heavily employed academics (especially demographers) in the elaboration of population policy and does not encourage work on issues that may be construed as politically awkward. Mexican researchers at several organizations told the author that their managers had communicated a preference for them not to study abortion-related issues.[86] Furthermore, limited statistical data, its poor quality and the illegal status of abortion have led many researchers to pass over the subject. Many are also ambivalent about it.

Researchers have, however, pointed to some of the costs of incomplete abortions and thereby exercised influence with policymakers and reform advocates. The IMSS family planning programme, the largest in the country, was estimated to have prevented 362,700 hospitalizations for incomplete abortions, as well as 3,556,700 unwanted pregnancies, and freed up US$2 billion for other expenditures between 1972 and 1985.[87] A more recent study examining the costs of alternative treatments for incomplete abortion confirmed that MVA is a more cost-effective means of patient management than sharp curettage, prompting IMSS to extend the use of MVA across its health care system.[88]

Journalists have publicized the issue of abortion. Arguably, journalistic opinion has shifted in favour of abortion law reform,[89] but media coverage still shows self-censorship related to the government's unwillingness to discuss abortion. Even if many criticisms surface, the state still holds *de facto* control over much of the Mexican media, particularly television, which promotes family planning activities through the social message-bearing 'telenovelas' (soap operas) but generally avoids mentioning abortion.

External influences

Feminists have still not developed significant transnational linkages that could pressure the government to reconsider the question of abortion, although any such alignments would be watched very carefully by the government. The subject of abortion was given scant attention at the Fourth Encounter of Latinamerican and Caribbean Feminists, a major feminist meeting held in Taxco, Mexico, in 1989.[90] Three years later, the first Central American conference on women's health (co-sponsored by the World Bank) called on public health specialists and women's groups to be centrally involved in debating and confronting the public health implications of abortion.[91] Participants also criticized regional governments for neglecting to do so. Frightened by such vigorous open debate about abortion, health agencies and governments ensured there would be less discussion of abortion at the follow-up conference held in Mexico in 1993.[92] In response, a committee of reform-minded researchers and activists sought to secure implementation of both sets of conference resolutions, and to provide information that could facilitate a new legal initiative on abortion. The group advised the Health, Justice, and Population and Development Commissions of the Chamber of Deputies, but proved unable to affect any significant change before the end of the *sexenio* (the six-year presidential term).[93]

The US 'Mexico City policy' discouraged the use of any money for research on abortion, although it did not expressly forbid such work. But, prior to its annulment in 1993, the diffusion of discourse on reproductive rights began to provide a new opportunistic focus for reform advocates and activist researchers. GIRE has used this rubric to rearticulate and strengthen women's demands, viewing abortion rights as part of a broader reproductive health agenda. IPAS has provided assistance in the management of incomplete abortion, paving the way for MVA equipment to be cautiously extended to larger IMSS hospitals. The Population Council, the Ford Foundation, and the John D. and Catherine T. MacArthur Foundation have supported reproductive health work, whereas the National Institute of Public Health's reproductive health programme has tended to avoid abortion. These developments notwithstanding, research findings have been poorly disseminated, institutional coordination between the various programmes and groups has proved elusive, and the state has paid little attention to their concerns.

BARRIERS TO REFORMING ABORTION POLICY

Many reasons explain why abortion does not command higher agenda status and why revisions in abortion policy are not being more seriously studied at the national level. They include the strong opposition of church-based groups and conservative sectors, the failure of potential reformers to successfully press the issue, and the lack of a societal consensus over abortion. A full explanation for this state of affairs, however, must take into account other structural impediments to policy reform. This is illustrated by the failure of feminism to find a niche within Mexican political culture, which lacks a tradition of issue mobilization and citizenry participation in debates, and remains heavily male-centred. The discussion below focuses on five sets of obstacles: women's marginalization; the low priority given to health matters, particularly to women's reproductive health beyond a rather narrow definition of family planning; cultural rationalizations of the personal dilemmas posed by abortion; the lack of research documentation; and a series of political obstacles.

The ability of women to transform their realities is impeded by cultural attitudes about sexuality and gender roles internalized by most men and women. This situation is made worse by the alienation of women's groups from the socio-political arena and inadequate societal and governmental attempts to improve their status. For example, in the early 1990s, the state resurrected the National Commission for Women earlier created for the 1985 women's conference in Nairobi. However, it remained an office without a budget, clear functions or authority, unable to develop public policies for women, let alone tackle sensitive issues such as abortion. Such marginalization is as crucial in understanding why there is no innovative reform of abortion policy as is the influence of Church-based opposition. Mexico remains a very male-dominated society; even if some influential politicians want to enact change, the indifference of the majority can be glossed over and rationalized away as Church opposition.

Mexicans do not think of health issues as politically important and, besides, there are more significant health problems than abortion. The state has tended to pay lip-service to women's health problems, despite having instituted its family planning programme under a rhetoric that stressed individual choice, equal rights, the promotion of health among women and children, and avoidance of unwanted pregnancies and illegal abortions. This helped defuse potential criticism, denied Church involvement in policy formulation, and disguised the programme's demographic objectives. But whereas the concept of 'population' was broad when the state first defined rapid population growth as a problem and adopted family planning as a solution, this dominant paradigm within the official discourse of population later overruled such concerns as the reduction of abortion. By the late 1980s pressure from donor agencies, NGOs and feminists had instilled a new sensitivity to issues of gender, informed choice and quality of care. However, family planning programmes have tended to employ only demographic targets, viewing women as producers of unwanted children and potential contraceptive acceptors rather than as empowered decision-makers and clients. Governmental, technical and popular discourse on the subject has been preoccupied with the absolute number of births and the annual growth rate rather than improvements in the health, well-being and social status of women. Likewise, family planning has been accepted by most people out of economic necessity rather than out of concern about women's health or their self-autonomy. This makes it difficult to accept abortion for public health reasons.

There are certain culturally accepted ways of resolving the contradictions posed by abortion which have reduced the visibility of the phenomenon. Anthropological data from several semi-rural and rural Mexican communities shows that abortifacients have been redefined as medicines for keeping a woman's period regular.[94] This conceptual ambiguity helps rationalize the termination of an early pregnancy in the face of religious injunctions. Past neglect of the topic by researchers has additionally contributed to its oversight. Documentation ceased once the existence of illegal abortion and the preventive effectiveness of family planning activities were pointed out, with research interest having only recently resurfaced.

A series of political obstacles blocks more serious consideration of abortion law reform. These barriers include the lack of political incentive for policymakers to carry out reform; the fear of opposition and the high priority given to system maintenance; the nature of governance, especially the centralization of power and the limits on political participation; and the use of the issue for other ends. Successive governments have explored public opinion on abortion and appear to have found the matter too sensitive. Elite and societal consensus on the subject is lacking, and there is no obvious political advantage to changing the status quo. Whereas Mexico's young technocratic rulers have found important constituencies of support for their reforms on free trade, opening up the economy, privatizing land and improving relations with the USA and the Catholic Church, there has been no politically significant sector calling for the legalization of abortion. The perceived threat of a reaction to such a move from conservative circles has contributed to government inaction, because of the high priority placed on maintaining political stability which is equated with the ruling party's continued hold on power. Accordingly, policy alternatives that might disrupt system equilibrium are unlikely to be seriously considered or followed through.

The influence of Church-based opposition has been overstated in the past, providing secular authorities with a convenient excuse for ignoring the consequences of unsafe abortion. Nevertheless, the rejection of anti-clericalism as an outdated state ideology legitimized religious-based opposition to the operation and emboldened the Church hierarchy to speak out, as evidenced in the controversy over abortion in Chiapas. This legal initiative may have fitted the image of the government's modernization programme, but it also prejudiced the pursuit of improved church–state relations. Mexican elites tend to comply to a social Catholicism, even if they are not Catholic themselves.

Groups seeking to liberalize abortion law are further impeded by the low levels of mobilization and political participation, and the scepticism and cynicism shown towards a political system which is only slowly becoming less authoritarian and more open.[95] It is likely that, given the corporate structure, the state would want to negotiate any policy change to preserve the impression of social harmony. This may have been possible in 1976 when the government commissioned an expert study of abortion and opened up debate on the subject, shortly after it had turned around its population policy. However, the policy window was closed off as the *sexenio* neared its end. It remains difficult for opposition parties to successfully pursue this issue, though their leverage increased after midterm elections in 1997 forced the ruling party's President to negotiate with them on key issues.

Mexico retains a highly centralized bureaucracy and political hierarchy, with the President enjoying considerable latitude and discretion in policymaking. Despite elite awareness of the existing problems associated with abortion, fear of being ostracized or demoted means that nobody is willing to support major policy changes without 'linea', or clear authority from the top. Significantly the hard-line Governor of Chiapas who presided over his state's initiative to legalize abortion never publicly mentioned the subject after being appointed as Interior Minister. This suggests that the President enforced silence on the subject and that promotion of the issue, and prospects for policy changes, will depend primarily on the President's belief and his political assessment rather than on such factors as the level of specialist knowledge provided to lower-level decision-makers.

For now, the issue of abortion is not judged sufficiently pressing to merit action. In fact, it has been used as a political game for different ends by various political circles. Powerful conservative groups, supported by PAN, have used it to exert some political influence against PRI. The left used the controversy over the move to legalize abortion in Chiapas as part of a tactical game to oust the authoritarian State Governor and treated abortion *per se* as a secondary issue. Many leftist deputies soon backed away from the measure, ostensibly because abortion was decriminalized for demographic reasons. They preferred to exploit an opportunity to discuss broader political issues, particularly non-democratic behaviour, rather than concrete matters of public policy. The dispute also showed that political parties will transfer their attention as soon as a new issue arrives. The federal government postponed discussion and defused the problem by claiming it was the governor's initiative and shifting the issue to the National Human Rights Commission.

The campaign promise made in 1982 by President Miguel de la Madrid to review abortion law was dictated by circumstances rather than benevolently motivated. In the midst of a major economic and legitimation crisis, he could not reproduce the clientalistic set of relations that traditionally allowed normal government, prompting gestures to women's groups demanding such a change in return for their support. The initiative was closed off once its detractors rallied more strongly than did its supporters. The Chiapas initiative likewise came from the ruling party, as did the resolution to suspend the law; the left was no longer in the forefront to liberalize abortion laws. Given that Mexican state congresses generally act as an extension of the executive branch, the initiative may have been an attempt by the President to test the waters for a similar move nationally. It is hard to believe that a state government controlled by the ruling party would express itself independently on such a complex political issue. Abortion can also be used as a political issue to rally support from those concerned about 'family values' and to secure Church favour, and bargaining chips in the process, by preventing a liberal law on abortion being enacted. Such political games underscore the complexity of the policy-setting on abortion and the reluctance to open it up to scrutiny, leaving discourse to be conducted through subtle and indirect channels. It also makes for a stew of apparent contradictions.

CONCLUSIONS

Whereas information on resort to abortion is extremely sparse, the potential magnitude of existing problems is reasonably clear. For women, abortion has long been a major cause of ill-health, including death, that was hidden from public discourse. The pretence that it did not happen because it was outlawed merely perpetuated the problems, although such a contradiction may not seem at all strange or troubling to much of society.[96] In contrast to their active leadership in providing family planning services, which has helped reduce abortion, government elites have passed over the problems associated with legally restricted abortion. Indeed, abortion first emerged as an issue when the state defined rapid population growth as a threat to development efforts, and only then to help justify the introduction of family planning.

Abortion has been debated periodically over the last two decades. In between such points in time, the issue of abortion seems to have vanished underground rather like the practice itself, with policymakers seemingly aloof to the circumstances surrounding it. Until the controversy surrounding a regional initiative to reform abortion laws in late 1990 demystified the subject further, discussion of abortion was largely confined to elite and technocratic circles. This was due to the continued strong presence of Catholic and traditional social values, as well as the closed nature of the policymaking system. Governmental ambivalence and past indifference over the question of abortion can only be understood within this context.

Whereas societal and elite awareness of the social and health problems associated with the existing situation have increased, the government perceives no compelling political reason to initiate policy change. Any such move is seen as a liability at present because of the opposition it would provoke among conservative groups. It would be naive, however, to conclude that this situation is due almost wholly to the Church's power, which has been limited politically to date. Besides, the potential has existed to change abortion policy, and governments are known to have heard and weighed arguments for doing so, for some time. Although the Church's position is now strengthened by its new *entente* with the state, it may still be unable to assert its views as strongly and effectively as it would like.

The question of abortion policy reform has also been funnelled away from agenda status by a 'system of bias' that limits serious consideration of policy alternatives judged by the government to be at once too disruptive, controversial, and bearing insufficient political gain. This is not to say that such a policy shift will not occur one day. For example, new discourses, such as reproductive rights, may come to challenge this status quo. Conflict over abortion is likely to be more difficult to contain as society becomes more open and as women develop greater choices and secure more influence. Without more fundamental political and social change, only minor efforts will be made to confront the reality that abortion is a greater problem than it need be. The country's leaders are unlikely to want to precipitate one more divisive social controversy and a bitter conflict with Church-linked groups, the Mexican hierarchy and the Vatican over abortion. A thin shroud still covers considerations of abortion, even though the veil of secrecy about it was lifted some time ago. This is why, for the time being at least, new ways of negotiating the hidden reality of abortion are unlikely to advance much further.

4 Abortion in Poland: Peering into Pandora's Box

'A nation that kills its own children is a nation without a future.'[1] With these words, Pope John Paul II laid down the gauntlet to Polish parliamentarians after they had approved a liberal amendment to three-year-old abortion restrictions. These developments in the 1990s occurred only after sustained and bitter conflict during a momentous political, social and economic transformation. Apart from 'decommunization', or the purging of those said to have collaborated with the overthrown regime, no other issue during this period opened up such a Pandora's box as abortion. The Pontiff repeated his uncharacteristically harsh words during his seventh papal trip back to his homeland in June 1997, just days after the Constitutional Court had struck down key provisions of the newly liberalized abortion code and instructed parliament to review it within six months.

Abortion policies in Poland have, in fact, changed radically in the post Second World War period. The legal position itself has been revised from restrictive to permissive and back to restrictive; it was then moderated once more until the high court had invited another legal change. A very liberal abortion regime had been introduced four decades earlier following the lead taken by the former Soviet Union in 1955. Poland shortly thereafter made abortion legally available practically at the request of a woman, and the procedure promptly became a primary means of fertility regulation. Similar developments occurred in most of the other European socialist countries, although pronatalist concerns later led several of them to re-enact restrictions on abortion.[2] In 1989–90 the dramatic collapse of the socialist order led not only to the transformation of political and economic arrangements, but also to a review of social policy, including the question of abortion, throughout East Central Europe.[3] In general, these countries have retained liberal grounds for obtaining a legal abortion, even after they had engaged in a wholesale restructuring of the laws and institutions of communist

110

regimes. Romania, Bulgaria and Albania legalized abortion on broad grounds, casting aside restrictions that were seen to cause high rates of maternal morbidity and mortality. Elsewhere, struggles developed between those who considered easy access to abortion services as a freedom that should be preserved and those who regarded this as yet another grave error of communism that had to be reversed. Sharp differences emerged in Hungary, Lithuania, the Czech and Slovak republics and in the two Germanies both before and after unification (1990) over what should be the law on abortion. Relatively liberal provisions were maintained, if not quite as wideranging as before. At mid-decade, therefore, liberal abortion laws prevailed across East Central Europe except in Poland, where deeprooted controversy over abortion has proved far more difficult to resolve.

This chapter attempts to clarify how and why a complete reversal in abortion policy took place after Poland had enacted one of the most liberal statutes in the world. The chapter also describes how the newly enacted restrictions on abortion themselves came to be challenged, and considers the implications of these policy changes over time. It explains the evolution and construction of Poland's abortion dispute, which has become as deeply embedded and divisive as that in the United States. Greater attention is paid to the move to restrict abortion (1989–93) as worldwide, it has proved very difficult in the modern period to ban abortion again after the procedure has been legalized. Moreover, this phase of conflict presaged the abortion dispute surrounding the 1994 UN International Conference on Population and Development. Indeed, participants in Cairo might have more readily anticipated that abortion could become the flashpoint of the meeting had they followed events in Poland carefully.

For over half a century, abortion has been a sensitive issue in Poland, caught up between competing belief systems and institutional forces. The communist state saw a liberal law as an instrument to confront the growing power of the Catholic Church, its ideological nemesis. With the fall of the regime in 1989, the episcopate sought a legal ban on abortion due to its doctrinal opposition to the procedure and as part of a strategy to reassert its hold over its followers and strengthen its role as an institutional actor. This furthered the Pope's broader plan to recreate moral rules for postcommunist societies and to promote a Christian revival. The Church in Poland had emerged from its epic struggle with communism as the only viable national institution and as an unquestioned source of moral strength. John Paul II himself came to personify Church and nation. While politicians dithered on the future shape of Europe, the Holy See positioned Poland as the heart of Europe, its spiritual centre and fountainhead for re-energizing the continent's faith. By restricting access to abortion, the Polish Church and the Vatican sought to establish a precedent for the former socialist countries of the region, and for developed and developing nations alike.

In the process, the intensely contested issue of abortion came to symbolize a wider dispute about the role of the Church in public life and the character of the future Polish state. The Church-sponsored initiative did not secure majority support among the public, even though 95 per cent of Poland's 38.6 million people are baptized Catholics.[4] This mirrored the apparent paradox of a high abortion rate coexisting in a society with a very high level of adherence to a Church that holds abortion to be a grave sin. Nevertheless, the Catholic Church's historical role as custodian of the nation is most significant. Having survived two centuries of often brutal foreign domination, the Church provided the umbrella that brought diverse social sectors together to the scene of a great triumph at the end of the 1980s. Once there, the Church turned triumphant. It had never forgiven the discredited regime for legalizing abortion, a measure ostensibly enacted out of concern for women's health but one the Church saw only as a direct affront to its teaching and, not without reason, as a weapon in the conflict between Church and state. However, abortion had become widely used for birth control purposes, chiefly because of a deficiency of contraceptive choices, with more reliable methods especially lacking. In such circumstances, a newly enacted ban on abortion would significantly affect the options by which women could control their fertility. The ensuing restrictions and the process by which they were adopted antagonized many people and church–state relations remain the source of much angst, a decade into democratic rule.

Poland has received worldwide attention in recent years. It gave rise to John Paul II, one of the most charismatic Popes ever, and to Solidarity, one of the most important social movements of the twentieth century. It spearheaded the democratic revolution in East Central Europe, the setting of one of the world's most significant economic experiments. Since 1989, Poland has also been the battleground of a major conflict over abortion that remains closely followed by the international media. This dispute has been a critical test case for John Paul II and for the Catholic Church in Poland and elsewhere. Many politicians invested heavily in this issue which is fundamental to women's and family planning groups and, more generally, to the causes of women's rights and family planning in Poland, East Central Europe and beyond. The conflict has also been a test for a fledgling democracy forced to resolve a highly controversial issue at a time of many pressing social, political, economic and psychological problems. The 1993 law fulfilled a longstanding goal of the Church, but proved a short-lived and Pyrrhic victory. It neither reduced existing problems linked to abortion and unwanted pregnancy, nor resolved the dispute surrounding the question of abortion. Controversy continued, following the liberalization of the law and after these amendments were declared unconstitutional and subsequently reversed. Indeed, both the underlying problems and the conflict concerning abortion persist with an intensity unimaginable before Poland entered systemic change, with no apparent end in sight.

ACCESS TO ABORTION SERVICES IN HISTORICAL PERSPECTIVE

Changes in Poland's abortion laws and policies, as well as in their interpretation and enforcement, have defined access to abortion services, affected the demographic and health profiles of abortion and shaped recent debate. The 1932 Penal Code allowed physicians to perform an abortion if a pregnancy resulted from a criminal offence or gravely threatened the health of the woman.[5] This was a relatively liberal policy for the period, although physicians often denied services because of their personal values. In 1956 a new law permitted abortion on socio-economic grounds, and its implementation was entrusted to physicians.[6] The law was qualified almost immediately by the Minister of Health, and again in 1959, when a woman's application alone became accepted as sufficient grounds for the procedure. No gestational age was specified as a legal time limit, leaving the matter to the discretion of physicians. Abortions were to be provided free in state health centres and, to help meet demand, on a fee basis in ambulatory facilities set up by medical cooperatives and in licensed private clinics, where they tended to be performed quickly and anonymously. In short, abortion became effectively available on request under the indication 'difficult living conditions'. However, many women sought abortions privately at a price and would seldom admit to doing so, with a large number of physicians profiting from women's misfortune.

Access to affordable abortion services became restricted in 1990. Three medical opinions and a consultation with a state-approved psychologist were needed to authorize a request. Physicians were also allowed to refuse to issue the certificate needed for the procedure when it was requested on nonmedical grounds.[7] State hospitals were then told to charge the equivalent of US$80, about one-third of the average monthly family income, for abortions obtained on such grounds.[8] A new medical code of ethics took effect in May 1992, forbidding physicians from performing abortions unless a pregnancy had resulted from a criminal act (taken to mean rape or incest) or threatened the woman's life or health.[9] The cost of a private abortion reportedly tripled to between $250 and $800, the latter figure several times the average monthly salary, as many health facilities stopped providing abortions.[10]

The law passed in 1993 permitted abortion only in public hospitals and only in cases of a serious threat to the life or health of the woman, as certified by three physicians; if her pregnancy resulted from a crime that had been reported to the police; or if prenatal tests, allowed only if there was good reason to suspect foetal defects, showed the foetus to be severely and incurably malformed.[11] Those performing illegal abortions could be imprisoned for two years, except women terminating their own pregnancies. The state was required to ensure sex education in schools and access to methods of 'conscious procreation', a clumsy euphemism brought on by a political compromise and one that not everyone equated with contraception.

These sections of the law remained ignored while newspapers in major cities advertised abortion services, some overseas, using readily understood codewords. The Justice Ministry reported that not one of the 53 cases of alleged illegal abortion investigated in the law's first year resulted in a conviction. Further, there were 30 cases of false denunciation, and one physician suspected of performing an illegal abortion committed suicide.[12] The medical ethics code was moderated in late 1993 to urge physicians 'to try to keep the life and health of a child before its birth' and *de facto* permitted prenatal testing again.[13] By then, an abortion cost up to five times the average monthly income.[14] Attempts to prosecute those accused of unlawfully terminating pregnancies or organizing trips abroad for women wanting abortions ended in acquittals and suspended sentences.

The law was amended in 1996 with the new regulations going into force in January 1997.[15] These allowed abortion up to the twelfth week of pregnancy if pregnant women faced major financial or personal difficulties, provided they underwent counselling and a three-day waiting period. The measure did not specify eligibility criteria so that its implementation could be subject to broad interpretation. It also provided for subsidized and improved access to modern contraceptives, as well as sex education in schools. Physicians, permitted once again to conduct abortions in private clinics, frequently cited the conscience clause in the medical ethics code and refused to carry out terminations in state hospitals, though many would charge from $200 to $350 for performing the procedure privately. Five months after adoption of the liberal amendment to the law, the Constitutional Court struck down its major provisions when it ruled that abortion violated the nascent democratic order, thereby ensuring that the issue would be revisited again after the 1997 parliamentary elections.[16] The more liberal provisions remained in effect until December that year, at which point the stricter 1993 law was reinstated.

THE MEDICAL DEMOGRAPHY OF ABORTION

Liberal abortion legislation in Poland had far-reaching consequences. More people came to rely on abortion as a method of birth control than would have done so had modern contraceptives been more widely available and their use and benefits better understood. For the late 1970s and the 1980s, estimates of the incidence of induced abortion ranged from 250,000 to 620,000 annually. This is at least two times higher than the roughly 130,000 cases suggested by official records, which tended to include only abortions registered in state health centres. While there is no certainty as to the exact magnitude of the numbers of abortions, owing to incomplete data, it is universally considered to be a mass-scale phenomenon.[17]

If prior to 1990 there were close to 500,000 abortions per year, as generally assumed, this implies a ratio of about 75 induced abortions per 100 live births. This is three times greater than incidence levels observed in the United States, where levels are high relative to most other economically developed countries. However, it is lower than in Bulgaria, former Yugoslavia, and especially Romania and Russia, where little use was made of contraception.[18] One estimate for the end of the 1970s suggests that in the absence of existing levels of contraception and abortion, the number of births in Poland would have been 108 per cent and 75 per cent higher respectively; the corresponding figures for France were 210 per cent and just 3 per cent.[19]

The number of registered abortions fell dramatically once the campaign to restrict access to abortion began, from 105,333 abortions (or an induced abortion ratio of 17.9 per 100 live births) in 1988 to just under 31,000 in 1991 (Fig. 4.1). The latter, totally unrealistic figure suggests there were only 5.7 abortions per 100 live births. The Ministry of Health reported only 777 abortions in 1993 (the first year of the new law), a slight increase in recorded miscarriages to 53,057, and 153 cases of mothers who had abandoned their newborn infants in hospitals. In 1994 there were 782 induced abortions of which 205 were performed to save the lives of pregnant women; 484 in cases of threats to the health of women; 19 for reasons of rape or incest; and 74 in situations where congenital defects were established.[20] In 1995, there were 559 legal abortions and 45,000 miscarriages recorded, but unofficial estimates suggested about 50,000 undocumented abortions with more performed overseas.

The author's interviews with gynaecologists and other specialists revealed that throughout the early and mid-1990s, some women in difficult living conditions could obtain an abortion under pretext. Hospitals were apparently attending to higher numbers of miscarriages, not all reported, with more women admitted on an emergency basis after having had an abortion provoked by a private physician. In one peri-urban hospital, the number of induced abortions fell from 74 in 1989 to 19 in 1990, while the number of reported spontaneous abortions rose from 48 to 85.[21] The restrictions on abortion did not prevent a fall in the number of births from 546,000 in 1991 to 443,000 in 1995 (Fig. 4.1).[22] The total fertility rate (TFR) first fell below replacement level in 1989 and reached 1.7 in 1995, the lowest birth rate recorded in postwar Poland. A government report conducted in late 1995 on the effects of the strict law stressed that its real dimensions could not be assessed. It also admitted that the regulations concerning sex education in schools and increased availability of contraceptives and assistance to mothers in difficult situations were not being observed.[23]

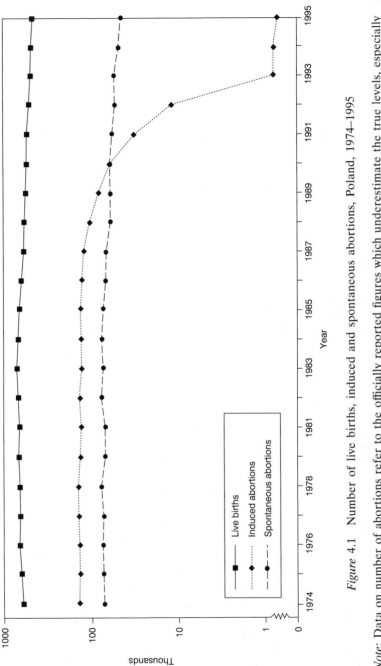

Figure 4.1 Number of live births, induced and spontaneous abortions, Poland, 1974–1995

Note: Data on number of abortions refer to the officially reported figures which underestimate the true levels, especially for the 1990s.

There are no representative data on the characteristics of Polish women seeking abortion. Until recently it was probably more common among those who had completed more years of schooling and among urban residents, although poorer women were likelier to abort in public hospitals. There was also a high, but unknown, proportion of repeat abortions, in large part because few women practised contraception after a previous abortion. The age structure of abortion seekers in Poland (and the former socialist bloc countries) has differed from that in the advanced capitalist countries, reflecting in particular a lack of effective contraceptive use among women who have reached their desired family size. Women aged 25 and older are thought to have accounted for about two-thirds of all abortions, with the highest rates among the 25–29 age group due to the postponement of or refusal to bear a second or third child. Among women aged 31 and over, induced abortions may have been more common than live births, irrespective of marital status, although the likelihood of having an abortion was higher among younger women.[24] This differs from the situation in more affluent countries, where the highest abortion rates are typically among younger and unmarried women (aged 20–24). In Britain and Scandinavia, for example, about half of all terminations occur among childless women. Information is lacking on whether the patterns described for Poland have changed as a result of either the policy changes introduced during the 1990s, or the profound socio-economic and political upheaval of the period.

Although the 1956 law helped protect women from the dangers of clandestine abortions, the quality of abortions performed varied widely. Several gynaecologists mentioned to the author that they knew of colleagues who carried out abortions without proper regard to the welfare of the women undergoing the procedure. Dilatation and curettage (D&C) was almost exclusively used, sometimes without an anaesthetic. Unlike the case of former Czechoslovakia, resources were never allocated for the introduction of vacuum aspiration, a technology deemed uncalled for by private gynaecologists and the chronically underfunded Ministry of Health. The scale of abortion-related complications resulting from outlawing abortion is unclear. However, the Ministry of Health confirmed three deaths during the first year of such rules, and even in 1990 a regional specialist had publicized the deaths of three women from self-induced abortions and let it be known that the National Chief Gynaecologist had asked him to alter their death certificates.[25]

A POLICY IMPASSE

The social context of fertility regulation in Poland

Abortion became a key method of fertility regulation in Poland and the other socialist countries of Europe. It came to be treated more as an alternative to contraception and childbirth than as an emergency act. It was readily accessible and widely known and understood, unlike modern contraceptives, which were often unavailable and of poor quality. Although the 1977 Family Survey in Poland showed that contraceptive prevalence stood at 75 per cent, the traditional and least reliable methods were the most widely used, particularly in rural areas. Among currently married women (aged 15–44) practising contraception, 35 per cent relied on calendar rhythm and 34 per cent on withdrawal, whereas only 15 per cent used condoms, 7 per cent pills, and just 2 per cent intrauterine devices (IUDs).[26]

At this time, survey data from Western European countries showed a large rise in the proportion of contraceptive users who had switched to more effective modern methods of contraception. Their societies were also beginning to approve of abortion under certain circumstances, with legal access restricted to specific indications and to the first few months of gestation. This ensured that the incidence of abortion would remain relatively low. In Poland and elsewhere in the Soviet bloc, the state in effect encouraged acceptance of abortion – which it had legally sanctioned and provided free of charge with minimal restraints – over that of modern contraceptives, whose production and distribution it monopolized but failed to promote.[27]

Faced with many demands for scarce funds, the state continues to ascribe very low priority to improving the quality of contraceptive care in the postcommunist period. The 1991 Fertility and Family Survey revealed that 28 per cent of persons aged 18–49 years having regular sexual intercourse had never used a contraceptive method, be it traditional or modern. Whereas only 7 per cent and 6 per cent of respondents had ever used IUDs and pills, respectively, 46 per cent had used withdrawal, 35 per cent calendar rhythm, and 32 per cent condoms.[28] Only one per cent relied on sterilization. Another 8 per cent had used the basal body temperature method, and 7 per cent the Billings ovulation method. Shortly after the new medical ethics code was approved in 1991, several Warsaw gynaecologists commented to the author that they were attending to many more women seeking contraceptive appliances and advice, while city pharmacists began to stock more contraceptives. However, there are no grounds to think that corresponding improvements have occurred in rural areas.

Family planning providers and survey evidence alike suggest that modern contraceptives are little used for reasons of ignorance, unfamiliarity, unwillingness to break Church edicts, lingering embarrassment, misinformation about their effectiveness and side-effects, and supply shortages. For example, oral contraceptives are little used because of limited availability and feared side-effects, in part linked to the high dosage levels of earlier versions. Many gynaecologists continue to consider hormonal contraceptives unsafe. In 1991 oral pills tripled in price after the state cut subsidies and withdrew several types deemed unhealthy. Sterilization is opposed by the Church and is uncomfortably linked in the popular mind with Nazi wartime excesses. Condoms are more widely used than any modern contraceptive, with their quality improving after the construction of a new plant in 1991 and the greater availability of imported condoms.[29]

Deeper institutional failures underlie these causes. Successive governments did little to demystify fertility control, sex education and reproductive health, or to provide objective contraceptive education and information.[30] During the communist era the inadequacies in contraceptive production and distribution could be compensated for neither by a nonexistent private sector nor through imports for which there was a lack of hard currency. Physicians found it simpler, less time consuming, and more profitable to recommend an abortion than to disseminate information or prescribe contraceptives that might be unavailable and about which they were often poorly informed themselves. The ready availability of abortion services may have additionally led to an abrogation of male responsibility for birth control. The Church has dismissed most contraceptives as harmful and abortifacient, reinforcing psychological barriers against their use. Greater awareness of the scale of abortion has influenced the Church to increase assistance to unmarried pregnant women and to promote natural family planning (NFP). Indeed, its family pastoral care service now oversees an extensive network of NFP instruction. While few teachers of the method are well trained and most are perceived as deficient counsellers,[31] many women apparently perceive rhythm as quite effective, even if its detractors dub it 'Vatican roulette'.

The socialist state did not develop a network of family planning clinics and it neglected the Family Development Association, the family planning agency it created in 1957. This token organization changed its name three times in a vain effort to come to terms with a difficult operating environment.[32] The agency was unable to combat its critics and the misperceptions concerning contraception. In 1988 its eight medical clinics and 25 family planning counselling centres served only 140,000 people. By 1990 it was a marginalized and almost bankrupt organization; its low profile and ineffectiveness led the International Planned Parenthood Federation (IPPF) to bring its affiliate together with several of the more activist women's groups to form a new Federation for Women and Family Planning in 1992.[33] The Federation promotes contraception and sex education. It also aims to keep the state tied to its new legal obligations in these areas – a tall order in a context where many oppose the provision of such services, and where there are many competing economic demands on state expenditures.

The acute deficiencies in housing and health services, widespread alcoholism, and low living standards have often been cited as contributing to the high incidence of abortion. Giving a child up for adoption is a complex and time-consuming procedure; orphanages tend to be run down. In the early 1990s, both state-run and Church-run shelters provided several hundred places each for needy single pregnant women. Such shelters rarely serve older married women who have completed their childbearing and who account for most abortions, and they are not oriented to assisting women several months after giving birth. Although senior bishops told the author that these services could offer assistance to all single mothers who sought it,[34] the aid offered remains inadequate to the scale of the problems associated with abortion. For example, the two Church-run homes set up by the future pontiff in Kraków, a city of about one million people, attended to just 1,000 women between 1974 and 1991.[35]

A legacy of Church–state conflict

In Warsaw, at one end of New World Avenue, stood the Communist Party headquarters. At the other end, tucked away on a side street, is the Primate's residence. In the postwar period, 'sex was treated as an instrument of battle, as a Trojan horse that rode from Nowy Świat [New World Avenue] to Miodowa' Street.[36] The regime would neither discuss social policy with the Church nor encourage open dialogue with society.

Following their attempts at persecution and repression, the state authorities finally reconciled themselves to an undefined yet substantial role for the Church, which increasingly championed the causes of human rights and pluralism and mediated between the rulers and the ruled. The Church formed an alternative hierarchy to the state, built on moral strength, not brute force. Under the statesmanlike leadership of Cardinal Stefan Wyszyński (from 1948 to 1981), the Church was strongly unified hierarchically and theologically.[37] Its authority grew with the election of John Paul II, who had earlier developed, along with other bishops and intellectuals, a social philosophy that stressed dignity and the defence of human rights. This cemented the Church's historic identification with the national consciousness and proved critical in securing the downfall of an oppressive system. In early 1989 the Church acted as a crucial broker in the 'Round Table Talks' that opened the door to political pluralism and the restoration of formal diplomatic relations with the Vatican.[38] These developments encouraged those who claimed that the 'communist' law on abortion should be replaced by a law in harmony with Poland's Catholic roots, rather than one that resembled the laws of an 'ungodly' West.

The debate in Poland about abortion policy is longstanding. The first two stages of discussion, in 1929–32 and in the aftermath of the Second World War, were largely restricted to elites. After the radical shift in the law enacted in 1956, two more phases of debate followed during times of relative political freedom, in 1956–58 and 1980–81. The transition to democracy in 1989 enabled opponents of the 1956 act to campaign actively for its reversal, culminating in the abortion law of 1993.

Adoption of the 1956 law followed a similar relaxation of abortion policy in the Soviet Union and formed part of the Polish communist state's ongoing confrontation with its chief ideological opponent. Church leaders could not effectively protest the new law, which passed without a meaningful societal debate. However, after his release from house arrest, Cardinal Wyszyński impassionedly proclaimed: 'We shall fight in defence of every child and every cradle as bravely as our fathers fought for the existence and freedom of the nation, paying a high price in blood. We are ready to die rather than inflict death on the defenceless.'[39]

The abortion issue was of interest not only to the Primate; it was also of concern to Bishop Karol Wojtyła, later better known to the world as John Paul II. Although there is no absolute verification, former associates attribute considerable credit to the then Archbishop of Kraków for helping to draft Pope Paul VI's 1968 encyclical, *Humanae Vitae*.[40] After its publication and the regime change in 1970 the Church intensified its opposition to abortion on several levels. The bishops addressed a strong message to the government on biological and moral threats to the nation. Their message declared that the law on abortion should be revoked and cited the high number of abortions performed. The bishops repeated these calls in pastoral letters and appeals throughout the 1970s.[41] Their criticisms were echoed in the expanding Catholic press and at the new marital counselling centres and premarital courses set up by the Church, which later began to talk with some hesitancy about natural family planning. However, religious, nationalist and medical opponents could not change the law. Also, abortion laws were not used as an instrument of state demographic policy, to be altered in step with changes in the birth rate.

A more heated debate took place in 1980–81, a period of great political turmoil and dispute regarding what was officially called renewal (*odnowa*). The Church reinterpreted this slogan of the time as the moral and societal renewal of the nation. The Church adopted a firmer stand against abortion and 'artificial' contraception, and fostered the growth of legalized lay anti-abortion groups. Moral arguments attained greater prominence than demographic concerns, which had subsided with the slight increase in birth rates. Nevertheless, the Ministry of Health did not enforce the new instructions it issued to limit access to abortion, and debate ended after the Solidarity movement was suppressed.

The Church broadened its anti-abortion activities in the 1980s, and by the end of the decade was ready to challenge existing legislation. It organized and supported various meetings dealing with abortion. Several seminars were held to mark the twentieth anniversary of *Humanae Vitae*, including one bringing together Catholic physicians and lawyers under the patronage of the head of the Episcopal Commission for the Family (which was formed in 1964). Participants petitioned parliament to repeal the 1956 law and give full legal protection to foetal life.[42] The same commission appointed experts to address parliamentary committees during 1988–89, and entrusted Catholic lawyers to draft a bill 'on the protection of the conceived child.' The Church explicitly took this as the starting point for reshaping Polish moral consciousness scarred by the previous regime. The stage was set for bitter controversy once systemic change began.

Despite the profound mistrust between Church and state, both sides tended to interpret moderate population growth as a sign of societal health. Although the state legalized abortion, which it characterized as 'an evil, though a necessary one',[43] it not only failed to make modern contraceptives widely available, but even introduced fertility incentives.[44] As a well-placed authority told the author, family planning was one of the transactions in the tacit understanding between Church and state, whereby the government extended some concessions and privileges to the Church in return for which the Church helped defuse the recurrent crises in the political economy.[45] The dramatic political changes at the turn of the decade made it even more difficult to provide sex education and family planning services. An elderly Minister of Education provoked fury when he linked sex education with the spread of AIDS and dismissed both as inconsequential: 'Sex education? I have never thought about it. I believe that there are more serious problems. Fortunately, AIDS is still only a marginal problem here.'[46] The situation did not improve after the government was bound by Parliament in 1993 and again in 1996 to reinstitute sex education in schools and improve access to contraceptives.

An ambivalent majority

Opinion polls that probe public attitudes about abortion are notoriously sensitive to the phrasing of questions and their field execution. For Poland as for the United States, attitude surveys reveal both a sharp polarization of opinion, and an ambivalent majority that is troubled by abortion but wants to maintain some form of legal access to it. One of the most reliable surveys, conducted in 1991, found that one-fifth (19.7 per cent) of Polish women aged 15–59 stated that they were categorically against abortion, and one-quarter (25.3 per cent) thought that women alone should be allowed to decide the course of their pregnancies.[47] The proportion in favour of a complete ban rose with age (27.3 per cent among those aged 50–59), whereas the fraction in favour of a woman's right to choose fell only slightly (to 22.5 per cent in the 50–59 age group) and was highest among those who were separated from a spouse (43.7 per cent) or who were dependent on social welfare to support one or more children (37.8 per cent). Those with fewer years of schooling, of higher parity and living in rural areas were more likely to favour prohibitions on abortion. The differentials became less significant in the event of rape or threat to the woman's health or life.

Opinion polls have shown that a slightly higher proportion of women than men supported a complete legal ban on abortion. A review of demographic surveys conducted between 1972 and 1984 suggested that about 50 per cent of all women thought that the Church's injunctions against abortion should be weighed in deciding on abortion.[48] More recent evidence extensively reported in Polish newspapers shows that seven out of ten people hold that the Church does not have a right to demand that believers submit to its teaching on the issue. Survey respondents routinely indicate stronger disapproval of abortion than actual behaviour suggests, reflecting greater relativism in practice. Since 1990, surveys consistently showed that about 70–75 per cent of adults believe the legal status of abortion should be settled through a national referendum.

In short, there is no societal consensus in favour of either strong restrictions or unfettered access to abortion services. While few people approve of abortion, most accept some mitigating circumstances. Societal attitudes towards the legality of abortion have proved relatively stable at the two extremes of opinion. Support for an outright ban declined somewhat during the initial course of the dispute and after passage of the 1993 law; but, by 1997, support began to wane for easier access to abortion as opponents of the procedure campaigned steadily to outlaw it again. All in all, the survey findings had little influence in this debate because everyone remembered how opinion polls tended to be falsified before 1989.

THE CAMPAIGN TO OUTLAW ABORTION, 1989–93

The political changes at the turn of the decade provided the setting for the most extensive conflict yet seen in Poland over abortion. Elsewhere in the region, the Romanian government that succeeded Ceauşescu's dictatorship immediately revoked a ban on abortion, as did the new Bulgarian and Albanian regimes.[49] Attempts to restrict abortion services proved unsuccessful in Lithuania and Latvia. Conflict over abortion strained relations between the two Germanies during unification. In 1993 the Constitutional

Court overturned a measure passed by the new German parliament, thereby preserving a dual abortion law system inherited from unification, with access being relatively straightforward in the east and more tightly circumscribed in the west. The law adopted in 1995 considers abortion during the first three months of pregnancy unlawful, but unpunishable so long as the woman first seeks counselling from an independent doctor. Despite some opposition, Hungary adopted a new law that retained moderately liberal provisions.[50] The sharpest disagreements occurred in Poland where permissive legislation quickly fell under sustained attack.

The Catholic Church applied moral, psychological and political pressure in an intensive campaign to replace the 1956 abortion law. The hierarchy's offensive was supported by the concerted action of many politicians who assumed the Church's mantle; the mobilization of anti-abortion groups; and the coopting of the medical sector. It began in early 1989 when Catholic deputies publicized a bill drawn up with the help of lawyers appointed by the episcopate. The bill envisaged an absolute ban on abortion, a three-year imprisonment for offenders, and a guarantee of the same rights for a foetus as those enjoyed by a living child.[51] Church leaders and other Church organs lobbied parliamentarians to support adoption of the anti-abortion law and called on parishioners to do the same. The outgoing communist government stirred media comment and ensured that the bill was submitted shortly before the first semi-free elections were held in June 1989, so as to split secular from Catholic members of Solidarity. The proposed harsh measure spawned a number of women's groups and pickets outside parliament, including defenders both of women's rights and of unborn children, but the reconstruction of the political system delayed discussion of abortion legislation for several months.

The Church-backed proposal became the basis for consideration of the matter in the senate (the upper chamber), which, after a stormy debate, approved a bill 'on the legal protection of the conceived child' in September 1990.[52] The bill stated that every human being has the legal right to life from the moment of conception; carried a sentence of two years for whoever 'provokes the death of an unborn child', allowed abortion only if it were needed to save a woman's life; and outlawed allegedly abortifacient contraceptives like IUDs and pills. A new wave of protest and debate broke out. The *Sejm* (the lower house) appointed a select committee, polled the public for its views, and took up a compromise nonbinding resolution from the Democratic Union (a party with strong Solidarity roots that generally favoured a clear separation between Church and state). The resolution urged a government ban on abortions provided by private physicians; a follow-up bill would have allowed abortion in cases of social hardship. House speakers confirmed to the author that these manoeuvres effectively postponed action until after the first free postwar elections were held in October 1991.[53]

The Church was furious with the Democratic Union's leadership, as indicated in a terse confidential letter sent to its chairman by the Secretary General of the Episcopal Conference,[54] and it pressured the government to further restrict access to legal abortion. A less restrictive bill was branded as 'communist' because many of its sponsors were members of the former regime.[55] After months of squabbling, the select committee recommended an even stricter measure than the Senate bill, permitting abortion only where the woman's life was at risk, restoring punishment for self-induced abortion, and banning in vitro fertilization treatment.[56]

A proposal to hold a referendum on the issue was successfully opposed by the bishops on the grounds that abortion was a matter of life and death, rather than of opinion or preference. However, the Church mobilized the faithful to sign letters and petitions when Parliament solicited public opinion on the Senate's legislative initiative, so that fully 89 per cent of the 1.7 million respondents (99 per cent in rural areas) favoured the bill.[57] A deputy from the Democratic Left Alliance (SLD), the successor to the Communist Party and the winner of most seats in the 1993 parliamentary elections, collected 700,000 signatures over three months to protest the bill.[58] Politicians were once again bombarded with mail addressing the issue of abortion.

Politicians allied with the Church redoubled their efforts to push through parliament a bill banning abortion in time for the Pope's visit in June 1991. Many Church sermons and statements during this period, as well as at other key points in the abortion debate, focused on the 'conceived child'. But as public opposition reasserted itself, the Sejm voted to postpone consideration of the 'anti-abortion bill'. The decision also reflected the composition of the 'contractual Sejm' created by the 'Round-Table' agreements: 65 per cent of deputies were holdovers from the previous regime, and most of these were supporters of abortion rights. In the freely elected but deeply fractured new parliament, the Christian National Union (ZChN) and the Centre Alliance parties, both supporting the Church, together won about 20 per cent of the seats. By early 1992, a sharply restrictive bill was again introduced in the Sejm, promptly countered by a proposal backed by the Women's Parliamentary Caucus. Also, the board of the Chamber of Physicians had approved by a slim margin a new medical code of ethics that forbade physicians from performing abortions except on narrowly defined medical or juridical grounds, under the threat of revoking their licence to practise. The code was loudly criticized for its content, for its variance with the law, and for the high-handed way it had been rushed through at an Extraordinary National Congress. The Minister of Health was not even sent a copy of the code.[59]

Parliament, left to resolve this legal absurdity, again considered two bills based on different philosophical premises and offering contradictory legal solutions. Meanwhile, over a million people signed a petition demanding a referendum, and public opinion responses continued to show most Poles in favour of maintaining legal access to abortion, though not on as broad grounds as had existed. The fragile coalition government was stretched to breaking point over the issue, but in January 1993 the Sejm approved a law that allowed abortion only in extreme cases.[60] The Catholic Primate, Cardinal Glemp, met with deputies moments after the bill was passed. He called it 'a step in the right direction'.[61] The measure was portrayed by the Christian National Union and the Church as a compromise because it fell short of a categorical ban, permitting amniocentesis when there were grounds to suspect problems with a pregnancy and dropping criminal sanctions against women who self-induced abortion. The new law ended the most bitterly disputed chapter yet in the conflict over abortion policy in Poland; however, it satisfied almost no one because it was poorly written and did not fully meet the demands of any one group. The issue seemed certain to resurface in the near future.

Organized resistance to a legal ban on abortion

In the early 1990s, groups that favoured maintaining legal access to abortion could not compete with the Church's strong reach at the grassroots level and in the corridors of power. Interest groups that formed after 1989 lacked an institutional infrastructure; those that had existed earlier, when associational life was controlled by the state, were unpopular. Both had to overcome the moral and emotional climate of fear that enveloped the abortion debate and prevented a more open discussion. Meanwhile, most people were weary, distrustful of collective action, and preoccupied with adapting to an unfamiliar world that included the spectre of unemployment. It is likely that a restrictive measure could have been adopted earlier had the proposed bills been more precisely formulated and had their supporters been more willing to compromise. There was also enough organized opposition from politicians, women's groups and the media to prevent passage of an outright legal ban on abortion.

Whereas some centrist politicians worked hard to temper the proposed restrictions and managed to postpone their consideration, the political left stressed that moral questions should be decided by individual consciences rather than legal stipulations. They insisted it was wrong to make political capital out of a deeply personal matter affecting women's bodies. They also argued that unless the economy was put right first, no other problems would be solved, including the creation of jobs and homes for those already born.

The Civic Movement for the Referendum coalesced public resistance to a highly restrictive bill. By the end of 1992, over a million people had signed the petition initiated by left-wing politicians and women's groups. Although not enough deputies backed the idea, the movement probably prevented a more restrictive law from being passed and secured for its organizers extra electoral support. Female deputies were few in number, but those from the centrist and left-wing parties formed a Women's Parliamentary Caucus. It submitted bills aimed at outflanking abortion opponents, collected signatures for a referendum and opposed attempts to remove contraceptives from pharmacies. The Democratic Union of Women, a political lobby closely linked to the Democratic Left Alliance, joined in these efforts. However, the post of Government Plenipotentiary for Women and Family Affairs remained vacant for almost three years after Christian National Union deputies ousted a minister they accused of failing to oppose abortion with sufficient vigour. The official fell out of favour once she sought to introduce the issue of limited birth control options into the debate about abortion.[62]

The position of women after 1989 in some ways became worse than under communism. One observer wryly noted: 'It is amazing to see how our rights have grown as humans but shrunk as women.'[63] In particular, women faced increased job discrimination during the transition years, a problem compounded by severe cutbacks in day-care centres and social welfare provisions. Many nationalists upheld the traditional model of a Polish woman, *matka polka*, the silent protector of the family and guardian of the nation, as symbolized by the cult of the Virgin Mary. Within this context, the abortion debate became a central concern to the new women's groups formed in reaction to the conservatives, who saw little role for women beyond the domestic sphere. However, they found it difficult to mobilize protestors after the initial rallies organized in several major cities against moves to restrict legal abortion. The new women's groups were small, dispersed, strictly urban and carried little political clout. Nevertheless, they made their voices known to deputies. They did so primarily through journalists and their involvement in petition drives and public demonstrations.

Feminist groups were equally ineffective because of their limited organizational capacity. They lacked resources, experience, unity and a clear vision. More fundamentally, feminism had not taken root in Poland. It was perceived as too similar to the bogus equality held out by socialism and by the Women's League, an organization set up by the old regime that retained a national structure but lacked legitimacy. The Polish Feminist Association could not correct this image problem because its energies, like those of Pro Femina and other women's groups, were sapped by the effort to keep abortion legal. Indeed, Polish women have yet to develop a consciousness of equal rights as known in the West. Their rights were formally granted, not struggled for. They remain sceptical of the value of political activism. Even if women were angered by the restrictions on abortion, they were too overwhelmed by urgent economic problems and daily survival issues to join the minority that did protest.

The Family Development Association limply defended legal access to abortion services. Tainted as a communist relic, its budget cut by the state and its very existence threatened, the Association was in an unenviable position; on the other hand, its members knew that if abortion was outlawed, ultra-Catholics would next try to restrict access to contraceptives. The Federation for Women and Family Planning spoke out more forcefully against the revised law after it had been passed. To this day, however, the Federation is little known, commands few resources and has no presence outside the capital city. The medical profession, meanwhile, remains weak as a lobby and divided over abortion, about which its vested interests have shifted over time.[64] Throughout 1989–93, few health care workers spoke of the need for access to modern contraceptives or of the dangers wrought by banning abortion. Only two professors of obstetrics and gynaecology publicly stated that the proposed restrictions served no medical purpose, the silence of others reflecting the mixture of intimidation and conformism that gripped their profession.[65]

The press was initially reticent to report on the abortion dispute, despite the social divisions, tensions and political conflict it generated. Editorial positions hardened as it became clear that there was little genuine attempt to find a societal consensus. The Church (like most politicians and much of society) found it difficult to come to terms with the multiplicity of voices in the newly uncensored press. It was particularly critical of press coverage of the abortion debate, some of which was openly anti-clerical. Television and radio, both monopolized by the state until 1993, offered little incisive comment and tended to report only on the parliamentary conflict.

An acrimonious debate

The abortion debate in the postcommunist period has been marked by hyperbole and an absence of compromise. One witness described the work of the 1991 parliamentary select committee that discussed the Senate draft as a 'complete waste of time, nerves and money.'[66] The committee quickly polarized into divergent camps, each with its own experts from different disciplines and backgrounds. Those convinced of their assertions and presenting their own truths felt there was no need to look at laws elsewhere. Poland was viewed as *sui generis*, with its own vast agenda of reform. The title of the proposed law on the protection of the 'conceived child' was at odds with internationally accepted terminology, but sat well within the context of the domestic moral crusade being waged.

Opinions differed sharply as to a suitable legal resolution of the issue and how best to reduce the incidence of abortion. Those working towards banning abortion projected the issue above all as an ethical-moral one, interpreted from a Catholic perspective, which invokes natural law and holds axiomatically that life begins at conception and should be fully protected. This teaching values sexual relations only within marriage and primarily for procreative reasons, and holds childbearing as the supreme mission of women.[67] All actions interrupting this set of relations, be it in vitro fertilization, 'artificial' contraception and especially abortion, are wrong. These views were buttressed by strong appeals to emotions, pronatalism and nationalism. The sanctity of life was to be defended, therefore, because of the biblical exhortation not to kill, Catholic social teachings on the family, the tragic experiences of Poland's disastrous losses under Nazism and Stalinism and its selection as the main site for executing Hitler's design for the Holocaust. It was said that: 'Totalitarian systems . . . had legalized the murder of innocent and defenceless children in the wombs of mothers.'[68] There had been enough killing already; now there was a need to show Europe the way. 'Even if Europe is heading in the opposite direction, we do not have to follow it.'[69] The way a society treated 'the unborn' was said to be a measure of its democratic standards.[70]

Those seeking to keep abortion legal likewise professed their opposition to abortion but did not claim to know when life begins. They asserted that equating the foetus with a human being, and abortion with murder, was a religious belief that should not be legislated in a democracy. It was argued that 'no state has the right to enforce these or other moral views by resorting to the knot, whip, or prison bars.'[71] The high levels of unwanted pregnancies and of abortion were primarily blamed on the Church's hostility to contraception and sex education. Many feared that the Church hierarchy would try to do away with contraceptives and institutional child care altogether. Abortions, they argued, would continue to take place even if legally banned, albeit at great health and financial cost, especially among the poor, leading to a new 'hell for women'.[72] Nevertheless, the Chairwoman of the Women's Parliamentary Caucus told the author that defining abortion as a matter of women's rights seemed vulgar and selfish in Poland, where women generally did not assert their legally granted equal rights and where the individual's right to privacy was not developed in the legal discourse. The proposed restrictions were best fought on pragmatic grounds since abortion was widely seen as a socio-economic problem and both state and society remained poor. The country could neither afford the burden of caring for the many injured women that she thought would result from illegal abortions, nor support the thousands of extra children that she expected would be born.[73]

Awkward realities were avoided or neutralized in the debate. Those calling for restrictions refused to consider that one could oppose abortion and at the same time object to a law that would make it illegal. The relevance of comparisons with the recently lifted prohibitions in Romania was negated on the grounds that the provisions there failed to recognize the personhood of the foetus, which lawmakers should defend, and because 'lex Ceauşescu' banning abortion was introduced as a tool of population policy rather than to defend morality. Hence nationalists and conservatives brushed aside as irrelevant the demonstrated failure of such restrictions to effect a sustained rise in the birth rate.[74] Likewise, they ignored the costs of treating the complications associated with unsafe abortion. The model provided by the Netherlands, which has the lowest abortion rate in Europe, was deemed unacceptable because that country permitted abortion, provided sex education and had a well-developed contraceptive culture. This included the use of IUDs and hormonal contraceptives, alleged to be abortifacients and threats to women's health. It was also argued that the costs of publicly financed legal abortions were very expensive and underreported. When the sordid conditions of Polish orphanages were pointed out, the retort was that they protected children from death. In such circumstances, it is unsurprising that the debate was poorly informed factually. The author was repeatedly told that 'numerical categories are meaningless, because moral categories are at issue here'.[75]

Those seeking to revise the strict 1993 abortion law pointed out that it did not stop the decline in the population growth rate and that fertility fell further below replacement level. By 1995 the birth rate had declined by one-third over the previous decade. Opponents of a legal ban on abortion used opinion poll data selectively, as did those seeking to outlaw abortion who also far more frequently misused demographic arguments. For example, presentations of the reported increased incidence of abortion and of fertility decline after 1956 failed to mention that very few abortions had been registered before the law was changed or that birth rates had started to fall earlier.[76] Such arguments can have a particular resonance in Poland, where interpretations of demographic trends, particularly of low birth rates, have often been infused in the popular mind with concerns about national survival. These sensitivities are linked to the series of invasions and demographic catastrophes inflicted by neighbouring aggressor states.

A large number of anti-abortion groups were formed across Poland, almost all under the auspices of the Catholic Church.[77] They included associations 'for the protection of life' and local foundations 'in defence of conceived life'. All these groups to varying degrees called for outlawing abortion; challenged the work of the state family planning agency and of health workers whom they accused of practising infanticide; and offered counselling and limited aid to pregnant women. In 1992 the deputy speaker of the Senate helped found the Polish Federation of Movements to Defend Life. Five years later, it affiliated 100 organizations and 50,000 people, many of whom would march in favour of keeping abortion illegal. These groups continue to denounce the 'civilization of death' in the affluent liberal democracies for permitting abortion and other perceived threats to the family.

The abortion debate offered an expedient arrangement for both the Church and conservative politicians. Many politicians adopted the issue as a means to build their own careers on the back of the Church, the country's only strong, national, and well-organized institution. Others feared the censure of a clergy whose endorsement could still be critical at election time. For some the debate was a means to identify political allegiances. Others thought the problem was more easily resolved and offered quicker results than pressing for political and economic reforms. They too tended to reduce this multi-dimensional conflict to a battle of symbols. As one politician noted of the party that pushed hardest for a total ban on abortion: 'For the Christian National Union, legal realism is less important than ideals.'[78] The Christian National Union appeared to attract the most support from the Church hierarchy and enjoyed a leading role in the shaky coalition governments from late 1991 to 1993. Afterwards, with right-wing parties under-represented in parliament, liberal-minded politicians ensured that the constitution approved by a referendum in 1997 carried no clause on the protection of conceived life. By then, former communist deputies in particular felt more confident about using the abortion issue to cultivate anti-clerical sentiments. The new constitution did, however, guarantee each person the right to protection of his or her life.

External influences on the debate

Western European and North American groups opposed to restricting access to abortion played a minor role in this debate. They were partly blinded by their own special concerns and experiences. For example, the North American women's movement has focused on women's professional employment and on abortion, whereas Polish women were granted substantial access to employment in the late 1940s and to abortion services in the 1950s. The IPPF and its French affiliate donated contraceptives, but Polish women's groups lacked the means to distribute them. These overseas groups and the US-based Catholics for Free Choice favoured the new Federation for Women and Family Planning over the Family Development Association, a lame survivor of the socialist era; but this preference undercut support for the only existing network of counselling centres that provided modern contraceptives, notwithstanding its inadequacies. The amount of domestic and overseas assistance provided to improve this situation remains minimal.[79]

Many of the photographs of foetal life displayed in Polish churches were supplied by groups based in the United States. For example, Human Life International, an organization promoting official Catholic viewpoints on abortion and sexuality, contributed various publicity materials. Much more importantly, the encouragement offered by the Pope made Polish activists feel fully prepared to lead their own campaign to ban abortion. However, most foreign observers interested in this abortion dispute felt that Polish lawmakers and the Church were reverting to bygone times. When President Lech Wałęsa visited the United States and France in March 1991, he was met by feminist and abortion-rights demonstrators who publicized the difficulties women faced in Poland. Deputies from the European Parliament appealed to the Sejm and Senate not to approve a bill that seemed anachronistic to the rest of the continent.[80] Such themes would soon be more actively championed within Poland itself as a new ruling coalition took office, built on the remains of the former communist system.

THE ANTI-CLERICAL BACKLASH, 1993–96

Another major policy reversal on abortion seemed likely after leftist parties were voted into power in 1993. The major victor, the Democratic Left Alliance, promised to lift the abortion ban, and the Women's Parliamentary Caucus submitted a liberal amendment to the law. All sides expected a new conflict. Nothing happened until May 1994, just after several ministries released reports critical of the new law. Both houses of parliament narrowly approved an amendment to the penal code, permitting abortion during the first 12 weeks of pregnancy in cases of social hardship. President Wałęsa the former Solidarity leader and a devout Catholic with eight children, vetoed the legislation, a move that reform advocates in the lower house failed to overturn.[81]

The governing coalition afterwards seemed intent to let the matter simmer in parliamentary committees, thereby keeping its options open and the issue under control. It was preoccupied with guiding the economy and building its own credibility, having won a two-thirds majority in the Sejm based on only 36 per cent of the vote, whereas one-third of the electorate voted for right-wing parties that did not clear the 5 per cent threshold needed for representation. The ruling alliance also delayed ratifying the Concordat codifying relations with the Vatican. Angered by this delay and that the leading challenger in the 1995 presidential elections promised to moderate the so-called 'anti-abortion' law, the bishops urged Catholics to support Lech Wałęsa, instead. The incumbent, still seen as the lion of freedom abroad but increasingly perceived as divisive at home, narrowly lost a vote that boiled down to personality issues and also reflected complaints about clerics meddling in politics. A new bill to liberalize abortion followed one month after the election of President Aleksander Kwaśniewski, a former junior minister during communist rule; but whereas the firmly anti-clerical Democratic Left Alliance preferred to ease restrictions on abortion, the Peasant Party (the minority partner in the ruling coalition) was split over the issue.

A second attempt to change the law occurred in March 1996 when the Sejm decided by a 95-vote majority to send for review by committee a bill that would allow first-trimester abortions for women in difficult personal or financial situations. The Labour Union, a small leftist party, initiated the bill on one of the few occasions it found common ground with the Democratic Left Alliance. Opponents of abortion demonstrated outside parliament and sent hundreds of thousands of protest letters against the planned amendments. Proposals to hold a referendum on the matter failed, as all sides feared an unpredictable outcome. The abortion dispute overshadowed all other political life that summer and in August deputies voted 208–61 to amend the law. The Senate overturned the measure, with deep divisions resurfacing among female senators. Defying the appeals of the Pope, another large petition drive and rallies in major cities and outside the legislature, the Sejm barely mustered the two-thirds majority needed to reject the veto. In November President Kwaśniewski signed the new measure which went into effect the following January.

Old socio-political divisions reappeared with a new vigour. The Church immediately condemned a move that Cardinal Glemp called

'a general licence to kill, aimed at children'.[82] Bishops said that
the new law was not binding in the people's conscience and many
hospital workers heeded their calls not to perform abortions. The
Polish Federation of Movements to Defend Life, better integrated
and organized than groups supporting easy access to abortion services,
staged pickets outside such clinics. Although right-wing parties could
not prevent the left-dominated parliament from liberalizing the law,
they reorganized around two non-parliamentary bodies, Solidarity
Electoral Action and the more populist Movement for the Reconstruction of Poland. These alliances used the abortion issue as a
mobilizing vehicle and vowed to reverse the legal changes if they
won the September 1997 parliamentary elections. The new head of
the revitalized Solidarity movement, which continued to receive
Church favour, called for a civil disobedience campaign whereby
those opposing abortion would withhold paying taxes and social
insurance premiums. On the other hand, the issue of abortion divided the centrist Freedom Union (the former Democratic Union,
the largest opposition party) into its Christian Democratic and social
liberal factions.

On the eve of John Paul II's longest papal pilgrimage yet to his
homeland and after bitter feuding, a new constitution was passed
that left open the issue of abortion and included both believers
and non-believers. Also, the Constitutional Court ruled that financial or personal problems were insufficient justifications for deny-
ing the right to life, 'the highest value in a democracy', and gave
parliament six months to reconsider the issue. The Pope's visit came
in the midst of an election campaign with rightist opposition parties seeking to supplant the secular leftists in power.

Though John Paul II sought to keep his spiritual message away
from politics, he inevitably spoke on the divisive issue of abortion.
His opening address praised the country's progress toward economic
and democratic renewal, and referred to the need to respect the
rights of each person, 'especially the most defenseless and weak'.
Several days later, he told a huge gathering that 'the right to life is
not a question of ideology, not only a religious right – it is a human right'. He also repeated his phrase that had become some-
thing of a mantra to the anti-abortion movement: 'A nation that
kills its own children is a nation without a future.'[83] Aware of the
political import of his words, the Pontiff added the unscripted words
to his sermon: 'Believe me, it was not easy for me to say this,
especially thinking about my nation, because I desire for it a future,

a great future.' His words helped ensure that parliamentary proponents of a liberal abortion policy would not be able to overturn the court's ruling before the upcoming general election.

BROADER VISTAS

The Pope forthrightly called the 1990 Senate bill 'a worthy initiative . . . [representing] a first step on the way to overcoming the evil inheritance weighed down with the stamp of totalitarian materialism'.[84] Despite relentless Church-based pressure on the Sejm, however, John Paul II did not receive the anticipated gift of the anti-abortion law when he came to Poland in 1991. Big crowds still greeted the Pope, but few Poles were prepared to assume their assigned role as the moral and spiritual vanguard in revitalizing Catholicism in Europe. Five years later, John Paul II stated that the lifting of restrictions on abortion reflected a return to standards of morality under communism. The Church's mission requires it to speak on ethical concerns, and the position of the institutional Church and the Pope on abortion is well known. However, as shown above, the major effort expended to push through a restrictive statute was not broadly supported by Polish society, including most practising Catholics; indeed, it provoked much hostility toward the Church and was, at least temporarily, reversed. So why was the effort made?

The first reason lies in the Polish Church's loyalty to the Polish Pope, a special source of national pride and an immense moral authority. The day after the Sejm passed the 'anti-abortion bill', the Primate left with other bishops carrying 'good news' to Rome, where the Pope commended their initiatives in defence of human life.[85] As a moral philosopher, Karol Wojtyła has held a longstanding interest in the abortion issue; as a bishop, he turned his attention to giving practical help to women with unintended pregnancies; as an archbishop, he helped shape the encyclical *Humanae Vitae*; as a Cardinal, he was one of its main defenders; and as Pope, he has continued to denounce abortion and to promote the protection of unborn life.[86] For many Poles, supporting the passage of a legal ban on abortion became a testimony of their fidelity to the Church and to the Pope's teachings.

Second, the campaign to reverse the abortion law was made part of the Vatican's strategic goal to re-evangelize Europe. The protection of unborn life, besides being a cause championed in its own right, also functioned as an instrument serving this goal, and Poland was to provide the model. Several senior Church figures told the author that they saw their task as setting a moral example for other countries – a noble task also signalling Poland's return to Europe. Indeed, John Paul II, a strong internationalist, had long been convinced of his homeland's importance for modern times and for Catholicism.[87] Christianity was held to have undermined communism, but the latter had left people morally scarred, as reflected by the oft-cited figure of some half-million abortions carried out in Poland each year. Liberal abortion laws were thought to have created a behavioural norm that fostered a callous and un-Christian disregard for life. The Pope further wanted to reverse the liberal trend in abortion policy that had spread to most predominantly Catholic European countries, including Italy (1978), Portugal (1984), Spain (1985; and 1995) and Belgium (1990).

The Polish Church seemed well qualified for these tasks in other ways. It had to be united and strong to resist communism, making it disciplined, pious and orthodox on doctrinal matters. It stood out for its condemnation of abortion and 'artificial' contraception over many years. Church leaders depicted abortion as a black-and-white issue to provide a litmus test of fundamental moral choices, mobilize devout followers and reinvigorate the religious consciousness of their congregation. Many priests still inadequately distinguish between abortion and contraception by modern means, and most believe that a 'contraceptive mentality' leads to the acceptance of abortion as a valid means of controlling fertility. Many also fail to differentiate sufficiently between legal and moral precepts, a confusion taken to its extreme by ultra-Catholic politicians.

Abortion assumed greater political salience as it came to symbolize an escalating conflict between liberal and Catholic world views. While the Church was not alone in being unsure of its relation to liberal democracy, it turned triumphant for several reasons. It had lost its ideological enemy, and many within its ranks wanted to confront the liberalism and consumerism that were replacing atheistic communism. Democratization and pluralism had appeared as ascendant secular trends, robbing the Church of its monopoly of institutional virtue and exposing it to social criticism. The Church, which wanted to reassert its authority, was initially encouraged to assume a greater public role by Poland's new rulers, who felt indebted to it. With no countervailing power, no postwar tradition of independent organization, and an uncertain political situation, the Church found itself in an institutional and power vacuum. The Church was numerically and politically strong, yet paradoxically feared a loss of influence and allegiance. It sought to reinforce its position through legal-political means, taking advantage of an opportunity less likely to be open later.

Most Catholic politicians and intellectuals were prepared to support some restrictions on abortion, but many of them privately criticized the anti-abortion campaign and the measures proposed by militant Catholics. However, no linkage was drawn between those seeking a categorical ban on abortion and those recognizing some extenuating circumstances. One Church-based anti-abortion group unexpectedly criticized the 1990 Senate bill for 'attempting to reduce abortion through legal means without even touching the causes'. It warned that the bill would become the object of political intrigues and called for a new initiative to 'defend life' through providing comprehensive help for the child.[88] The minority Evangelical Reform Church took a more pragmatic stand. It favoured concentrating efforts on contraception, sex education, aid for poor parents and ethical awareness, rather than forcing a legal solution that neither solved the problem nor, it was said, was consonant with Christian principles.[89]

The abortion debate led to divisions in the relations between clergy and society, exposed contradictions between declared and actual religious behaviour, and intensified debate about the Church's role in public affairs. It also disrupted political life, increasing popular disaffection with elites and institutions. Parliament was widely thought to have wasted time on the issue instead of managing the economy. Right-of-centre parties had found a cause but were seen as obsessed with it and too closely chained to the Church. Unable to take the lead in the transformation process, with their political programme and style out of favour, not one Christian National Union deputy was returned to parliament in the September 1993 election. Although economic considerations dominated, the vote was also seen as a strong indictment of the agenda and style of the Polish Church in general. The banner of 'triumphant Catholicism' was tattered.

Several senior Church figures tacitly admitted to the author that they may have made some errors. They insisted, however, that the episcopate had approached the issue correctly and that the Church's image had been tarnished by politicians who had used it as an instrument for other purposes.[90] It was implied that the ends justified the means. Lay Catholics and nonbelievers, rather than the hierarchy itself, had stressed the importance of imposing penalties on transgressors as part of the new abortion law. Nevertheless, the episcopate did appoint advisers, some from within its own ranks, who had suggested such measures. It had also strongly supported the election of Catholic-nationalist deputies and did not object when they inserted criminal sanctions into the various anti-abortion bills. The Pope did finally tell Polish bishops to steer away from partisan politics just after the new law against abortion was passed; but he also commended their anti-abortion campaign and committed them to continue to guard the moral order and remain the state's critical conscience.[91]

The bishops believed that by pushing the issue of abortion, they had inculcated a greater awareness of the 'unborn child' and had accorded legal protection to the foetus. Churchmen were convinced this would ameliorate, if not necessarily resolve, the social problem of abortion. Senior Church figures thought that abortion rates had fallen and that the 'abortion underground' did not resemble that extant before the mid-1950s. On the other hand, only a precipitous fall in reported hospital abortions was certain; and there remained some unease as to why the birth rate continued to decline even after terminating a pregnancy became all but illegal. The official redefinition of abortion was itself overruled three years later. Meanwhile, the Church is neither willing nor able to pass on knowledge about preventing unwanted pregnancy; the state continues to fail to do so; and non-governmental organizations face many barriers in filling the gaps.

Lawmakers relaxed restrictions on abortion in 1996. This radical policy shift renewed sharp conflicts, dividing both the population and even the ruling coalition parties. The controversy also re-energized anti-abortion activists and conservative groups. However, the revisions did not result in as far-reaching changes as might have been expected for women seeking abortions. About half of all state hospitals declined to perform abortions on social or economic grounds, and abortions obtained privately remained costly. Support for the new liberal policy dropped slightly before the Constitutional Court struck down the liberal amendments ahead of the 1997 Papal visit. Earlier however, much of Polish society appeared confused, exhausted and divided by the abortion debate which continues to split most of those interested in it into roughly equal camps. It also exacerbates historical animosities between former communists and revengeful right-wingers.

More conflict was expected when a new parliament would revisit the issue following the instruction of the Constitutional Court, though few wanted to reopen the debate again. After four years of leftist rule, voters handed a strong victory to Solidarity Electoral Action, an umbrella group of over 30 rightist parties. It took office in a coalition with the Freedom Union. The new parliament, like the old, could have overruled the court with a two-thirds majority, but the victorious alliance had pledged to overturn the 1996 liberal amendments which stayed in force for a six-month grace period. In choosing not to do anything before the court's imposed deadline, parliament effectively reinstituted the former 1993 law in December 1997. Abortion would again be permitted only in cases of serious risk to the life or health of a pregnant woman, if a pregnancy had resulted from a crime, or in cases of severe foetal damage. Although pressure may grow on Poland to make its statutes more compatible with those of the European Union, it cannot be forced to change its law. The European Tribunal concerns itself with individual transgressions of human rights rather than with particular laws, which are difficult to appeal.

Very few organized efforts are currently being made to reduce the incidence of unwanted pregnancy in Poland. There may be a general presumption that the incidence is lower than it was in recent decades, not least because birth rates continued to fall after access to abortion services was sharply limited. This inference notwithstanding, official plans to develop sex education and make modern contraceptives more widely available were not implemented after the 1993 and 1996 legal changes. Very little Western assistance is being provided in these areas, or to improving the quality of abortion services legally allowed. At the same time, the state is too poor to provide significant social welfare assistance to women with unintended pregnancies or to improve the economic status of those who have given birth.

CONCLUSIONS

The abortion dispute in Poland is both longstanding and deeply rooted. It precedes the 1956 liberalization of abortion rules, a decision that was made under socialist rule without public debate.

Earlier, abortion was clandestine, not measured, and presumably common, though not as frequently performed as when it became a state-sanctioned procedure. Church leaders then spoke out against abortion, but their persuasive efforts could never reduce what was a widespread phenomenon among Catholics and nonbelievers alike.

With the downfall of communism, the Church mobilized its faithful and encouraged its political allies and the health services sector to restrict access to abortion, a cause upheld as central to the moral regeneration of society. For over four years, the ensuing conflict sparked great emotion, energetic campaigning and hostility during a time of major societal tensions that accompanied the rebuilding of political and economic systems. In sharp contrast both to the previous situation, which *de facto* permitted abortion on demand, and to the general retention of liberal abortion policies elsewhere in East Central Europe, access to abortion services was sharply curtailed through administrative decree and the intimidation of physicians. After two years of conflict, grassroots opposition to the proposed restrictions became harder to mobilize. Without a tradition of social movements, saddled by the double burden of domestic and salaried work, and suffering disproportionately from the economic crisis, few women fought to keep abortion legal. Advocates of abortion rights could not meet the challenge of triumphant Catholicism, although access to abortion services could be restricted only in steps. Eventually a near-total legal ban on abortion was enacted that remained in force for almost four years.

The state's provision of easy access to safe abortion services in the late 1950s led to an excessive dependence on abortion. This situation was exacerbated by the state's failure to make modern contraceptives more readily available and more familiar, when it alone was able to do so. Although the true magnitude of abortion is open to question, the precise level is less important than the recognition that it could have been – and still could be – considerably lower if contraception were more effectively practised. The incidence of abortion has most likely fallen since the late 1980s, alongside a shift to more preventive behaviour. In 1995, two years after the introduction of the anti-abortion law, the total fertility rate stood at 1.7, well below replacement level. This historic low underscored that the real magnitude of abortion was significantly greater than reported.

Churchmen had correctly identified the one state policy that more than any other enabled abortion to become a mass phenomenon;

but their diagnosis disregarded the urgent need to improve birth control options, overlooked the wider social causes of abortion and unwanted pregnancy, and ignored the broader reasons why so many practising Catholics disagreed with the Church's unconditional stance on abortion. Like the former communist regime, the Church and its political allies saw the issue in categorical terms and as a test case of their strength and influence. Leftist politicians persist in seeing the issue as an opportunity to mine anti-clerical sentiments. After several more years of conflict, the Democratic Left Alliance began to make political capital out of the attempts by clergy figures and Church-backed politicians to regulate women's access to abortion services. Abortion continues to be used instrumentally as a core means of shaping politics and as a crude index of the balance of power. The debate concerning it serves as a forum for discourse on the shape of the state and public sphere, the rule of law as well as other policy issues.

The Pope more strongly endorsed an anti-abortion bill in Poland than he has done in any other country; even when in Rome, his hand was still visible, waiting to hold up to the world a keenly anticipated model treatment of this issue. John Paul II had always seen the 1956 law as a national disgrace and as a threat to the health of women and the nation. Few of his compatriots listened to his appeals on this point when he made his triumphant return to Poland in 1979, even though 13 million people, or one-third of the population, turned out to see him in the course of nine days. Fewer Poles greeted him in 1991 than expected, but the frictions that had emerged were largely generated by the clergy rather than the Pope himself, and centred at least as much on the style of their interventions in public life as over their substantive positions. The same applied in 1997 when six million people attended the public appearances of the Pope. For John Paul II, the 1993 law and the overruling of its subsequent liberalization were bittersweet victories. Poland, the site of his most loyal Church that had just emerged victorious from its heroic struggle against communism, did not rise up to its scripted role as a showpiece for countries considering abortion legislation. Access to legal abortion services was severely limited, but religion had become an object in a political game, with the episcopate's judgement and actions severely questioned.

The 1993 law capped four years of tumultuous and divisive debate on changing Poland's abortion rules. It gave legal protection to the beginning of human life in preference to the autonomy of the woman, even if her health was threatened by pregnancy. Those who secured passage of the law slighted its preventive aspects. Indeed, missing from the debate that took place was any serious consideration of how to improve birth control options for women. The law lacked the support of most people and took insufficient account of social realities. It was rewritten three-and-a-half years later by a new government after communists turned social democrats gained control of parliament and then won the presidency. However, they did not institute promised policies to reduce abortion through improving health education and contraceptive practice. The Constitutional Court struck down the liberal amendments soon after they began to apply. A new ruling coalition effectively outlawed abortion again in December 1997, reinstating the 1993 law.

There is little indication that structures for delivering family planning services will be substantially improved soon. None of the major political parties are willing to make the necessary commitment, the state has its own fiscal limitations and other spending priorities, non-governmental organizations still encounter difficulties in their activities, and the Church steadfastly refuses to accept either sex education or modern contraceptive methods. Few people want to open the debate all over again. Yet another poorly considered and radical shift in abortion policy is bound to provoke sharp conflicts and perpetuate existing problems. The current polarization of forces over this issue greatly reduces the prospects for a compromise settlement. As with the story of Pandora's box, abortion continues to be the source of extensive and unforeseen troubles, with little hope yet for a peaceful resolution.

5 The Global Nature of the Abortion Debate: Realities and Prospects

This final chapter provides a more focused comparison between the three countries, concentrating on the more enduring aspects of the abortion debate and setting this discussion within a broader international context. As we have seen, total abortion rates in Kenya and Mexico are higher than in Western Europe and comparable to those found in the USA. They are even greater in Poland. Abortion rates will not decline further until contraceptive use becomes more widespread and effective. In all three countries studied here, issue mobilization over abortion is growing and is being facilitated by external linkages. This is generating pressure to reconsider and formulate new policies on abortion, a symbolically powerful issue. Nascent interest groups and liberal and left-wing political circles have clashed with the Catholic Church and groups spurred on by it. Although discussion about abortion is often poorly informed, the debate is moving from the private sphere to the public arena, slowly in the cases of Kenya and Mexico, rapidly in Poland. It is reaching agenda status as societies become more pluralistic and open to external interests, and states are finding it more difficult to contain the controversy and to reach an effective policy resolution. However, abortion is still not an agenda item for policymakers in most African and Latin American countries, even as it becomes better identified as a significant health and social problem. In Kenya and Mexico, for instance, the health dangers of unsafe abortion are now being tackled to some degree, but decision-making elites are unlikely to intervene more directly so long as they have little compelling political reason to act. Abortion remains stigmatized even as it is being demystified.

At the same time, poor countries must increasingly reckon with the pressures arising from the export of the abortion debate from Western countries, particularly from the USA, as well as from Rome. This study has underlined that dispute is being fuelled by the international links of the Catholic Church, of feminist groups, medi-

146

cal circles and family planning agencies. All these players in the abortion debate rely for their identity and financing to some extent on more affluent countries where such groups increasingly feel obligated to advocate their positions on abortion. As one feminist put it: 'We live in a global village. For abortion rights to be secure in one country, they must be secure in all countries.'

The abortion debate is spreading, but it is not carried on with the same depth in all parts of the world. Moreover, it does not take the same form across countries, reflecting cultural understandings of abortion at variance to those in North America or in Western Europe. And although the abortion debate is played out in more and more countries and in the world arena, it is not yet a truly globalized debate in so far as it remains a less salient concern in most poor countries, where women and men face a greater number of pressing problems and where there tend to be more barriers to organizing about this issue.

This study additionally shows the degree to which the Catholic Church has sought to extend its say on the way abortion is considered in different regions of the world. In Kenya and Poland especially, the Church has provided space for discussion of political change. In contrast to this liberating potential, it continues to lead a conservative movement on birth control, and specifically on abortion. Paradoxically, the Catholic Church has received little serious and sustained assessment from social scientists. This is all the more remarkable, given the Church's influence as a player in the abortion debate and its importance as a health care provider in many countries. Both Kenya and Mexico are pivotal countries in the Church's strategies to consolidate its position over abortion elsewhere in Africa and Latin America. Poland was intended to provide a model resolution of this issue not only for the fledgling democracies of East Central Europe, but also for the world. This analysis bears out that the strength and influence of the Catholic Church is not just a function of the organization itself, its official doctrines or other internal affairs. Rather, as with interest groups in general, it is largely dependent upon its strength relative to existing state and societal institutions. In addition, in all three countries, the Church has been associated with and spawned other groups with an interest in abortion. This is also an issue that national Church hierarchies themselves do not stress to the same degree, even though Pope John Paul II has made opposition to abortion a major theme of his papacy.

In Kenya it is increasingly realized that abortion has become a more common phenomenon. However, the attendant problems are still not receiving sustained attention from policymakers and there are a number of structural impediments to major policy reforms. Alongside this official silence, there is considerable societal confusion as to how abortion should be thought of and managed. It may well be a long time yet before the goals of reformers are achieved in a significant way, not least because government decision-makers are unprepared to make major changes in abortion policy. As in Mexico and Poland, the Catholic Church constitutes a significant presence in public life and a critical barrier to the adoption of more liberal policy.

In Mexico and Kenya public debate on abortion has only recently begun and is constrained by the lack of openness in the political process. Researchers have paid greater attention to other aspects of fertility regulation than abortion. However, Mexico has seen greater energies expended in changing abortion laws and policies, especially by feminist groups, with the Catholic Church and lay groups conspicuous in opposing such efforts. Although Mexican governments have taken note of the problems associated with the situation surrounding abortion, they have not explicitly addressed them. While the improved nature of Church–state relations would seem to preclude more substantive policy changes, there is limited evidence of a gradual decriminalization of abortion alongside improvements in the provision of such services.

The abortion debate in Poland is deeply rooted historically, unlike in Kenya and Mexico. Abortion became the primary method of birth control together with traditional contraceptive methods. The state failed to support either family planning or sex education. These remain neglected in the democratic era, at the start of which the Catholic Church managed to redefine abortion because it was the only strong, national and well-organized institution. Its powerful political presence and great respect is linked to the personal prestige enjoyed by John Paul II, who maintains a keen interest in his homeland. Three years after the adoption of a restrictive statute, however, another policy reversal occurred, checked by a high court decision the following year. Polish society has become sharply divided about abortion.

The Polish debate illustrates especially well how controversy over abortion can crystallize larger social conflict and serves as a kind of conjuncture of many different issues of social, economic, moral and political change. The resultant abortion debate has been particularly loud, emotional and polarized. As in Kenya or Mexico, the failure to make objective use of existing family planning and health data is apparent, though there is increased concern about the consequences of unsafe abortion. There is also greater awareness of the misuse of abortion for birth control purposes, and controversy about the circumstances that being this about.

THE DIMENSIONS OF THE PROBLEM

Our knowledge of the demography of abortion in Kenya, Mexico and Poland – as for most regions of the world – is incomplete and imperfect. Nevertheless there is no doubting the scale of existing problems. In Kenya the available data suggests substantial resort to abortion, although this does not yet significantly limit fertility at the aggregate level. Abortion is disproportionately common among adolescents in urban areas, as across much of Africa, and may be more widely practised by married and multiparous women than is presumed.

In Kenya and Mexico contraceptives are little used by youth. Young unmarried Mexican women are more likely to keep their unwanted pregnancies than their counterparts in most Latin American countries. The abortion rate for Mexican women in the older reproductive age-groups may still be higher than for younger women, but it has probably decreased as contraceptive practice has improved, particularly with the growing prevalence of sterilization. In Latin America abortion has had an impact on the fertility transition, which is far more advanced than in Africa. It seems probable that abortion rates in Mexico are lower than for most Latin America countries.

Both Mexico and Poland are 95 per cent nominally Catholic, but abortion rates are higher in Poland where abortion became a heavily relied-upon substitute for contraception and where fertility preferences are lower. In recent decades almost as many pregnancies have been deliberately terminated as brought to term. Abortion is particularly common among Polish women who have already completed their desired family size. This underscores the low rates of contraceptive efficacy, especially among those practising rhythm and withdrawal.

The health consequences of abortion are more significant than knowing the actual incidence in a setting where many abortions are poorly performed. In Kenya there is considerable ill-health associated with unsafe abortion, mirroring the situation across much of Latin America during the 1960s and 1970s. Complications from abortions that are self-induced or obtained from unqualified pro-viders contribute close to half of all maternal deaths in a situation where the maternal mortality rate is still very high. However, the ratio of badly to safely performed abortions remains undefined, as is true across Africa. In Mexico more so than in Kenya, abortion has become generally safer due to improved procedures, particu-larly the use of manual vacuum aspiration to manage incomplete abortion. Menstrual regulation services have been quietly initiated in Kenya, as in a number of African countries. Nevertheless, many preventable deaths continue to occur. Technologies that promise to make abortion practice much safer, such as the widespread use of vacuum aspiration, are likely to be brought into use only if legal and political problems are overcome.

The actual abortion rate, no matter how high, is not as import-ant as the process bringing it about. Whereas in Northwest Europe and North America it is to a large degree possible to separate abortion from contraception, this is less true in Kenya, Mexico and Poland, or indeed much of the world where people are less likely to use more reliable contraceptive methods. For example, the idea of family planning has long been accepted in Poland where, for several decades, contraceptive prevalence rates have been as high as in more economically developed parts of Europe. However, most people have been unable to practise birth control effectively owing to limited access to modern contraceptive choices, as throughout the former socialist bloc. Successive governments have failed to improve family planning services to this day, and the deficiencies are only partly being made up by a few NGOs.

Abortion is becoming more common in Kenya and elsewhere in Africa as the motivation to control family size increases. Modern contraceptive use is also increasing and will exercise a preventive role, but, like sex education, it is no panacea. Despite high overall levels of education, ignorance about human reproduction and sexu-ality remains widespread even in many industrialized societies, with contraception often improperly used, if at all. The experience of the USA, which leads affluent countries in adolescent pregnancy and abortion rates, shows how counterproductive is the failure to face up to the reality of adolescent sexuality and to wrangle excessively over its morality. While sex education was introduced earlier in

Poland than in most Western countries, and later on in Mexico and Kenya, the general tone of such programmes in all three settings is very cautious and prudish.

In Kenya, Mexico and Poland, a broad array of cultural, social and political sensitivities perpetuate abortion-related problems and make their discussion more difficult. These problems are not addressed by politicians preoccupied with maintaining support and control. At the same time, concerned researchers and physicians are worried about antagonizing politicians should they raise these matters, and women's groups are too weak to exert significant influence. The societal indifference and semi-official neglect is compounded by negative attitudes to female sexuality, a reluctance to re-evaluate gender relations, the lack of political participation and the influence of those implacably opposed to considering the broader context of abortion.

The Polish statute of 1956 predated the liberalization of abortion rules in North America and most of Western Europe by at least a decade, although there was always a disparity between the letter of the law and its application. Equally, longstanding legal restrictions on access to abortion services have been widely abused in Mexico and Kenya. Women seek an abortion irrespective or religious or legal injunctions, or their stated beliefs when not pregnant. Whereas problems may occur for those working on the margins of the law, legal sanctions are not strictly enforced in Kenya and Mexico. However, their statutes restrict access to safe regulated services, and the state spends scarce resources on caring for women with incomplete abortions and related complications. In all three countries the costs of treating such cases have yet to be satisfactorily quantified. Existing studies are methodologically flawed, so that their policy prescriptions receive little attention.

THE USES AND ABUSES OF DATA

In Kenya, Mexico and Poland abortion is widely condemned in public, but social and cultural objections to it may be weaker than is commonly thought. Opinion surveys show a profound ambivalence about abortion and policy options in Mexico and Poland, just as in the USA. They also suggest that most people favour permitting abortion on broader grounds, though not on request.[1] However, opinion polls are rarely a good gauge for abortion policy. Many who say one thing in a survey do not act the same way when confronted with a crisis pregnancy, as highlighted by Polish data. Furthermore, views on the morality of abortion diverge from those on its legality. Public opinion may prove more important in influencing policymaking as political participation increases, but in Kenya, Mexico and Poland it does not play as strong a role as in the liberal democracies.

The experience of all three countries shows that the absence of good quality data about abortion hinders the development of a more informed debate and encourages erroneous statements. It also makes decision-makers less inclined to review existing policy and deprives them of a more informed framework within which to consider policy options. All the same, enough is known about the dangers of unsafe abortion to guide decision-making. Instead, information from public health workers, gynaecologists, family planners and demographers continues to be overlooked by policy elites.

Clearly there are strong limits to the use of data. Religious and political conservatives, for example, often refuse to accept the need for accurate abortion statistics. In Poland they asserted that statistical data were manipulated and carried no meaning in relation to moral concerns. They also selectively interpreted demographic data, linked abortion to fears of population decline, and insisted that its incidence could be dramatically reduced through legal prohibition. Such wishful thinking and refusal to learn from known experiences of abortion bans ensured that debate would be poorly informed factually. Opponents of abortion could yet use statistics more effectively. This is underscored by the work of the Mexican group Pro-Vida. In the early 1990s it began to publicize the number of pregnant women counselled at its Women's Aid Center and the number of abortions this may have prevented.

Governments may fail to act on data. In Poland socialist planners did not heed specialist advice on how to reduce abortion through designing better quality family planning programmes. In legalizing abortion they apparently felt they had at once provided a means by which women could control their fertility and scored a point in their conflict with the Church. This indicates that the political process, including the ideological preferences and values of the ruling elite, can be a far more important input into the formulation of abortion policy than data or knowledge about the actual context of abortion.[2] Even assuming greater rationality, decision-makers are unlikely to consider policy changes unless the need is impressed upon them and sufficient data is transmitted and explained directly to them. This is more difficult to bring about for concerned publics where political participation is restricted and opposition to abortion is well mobilized.

More research is needed to improve understanding of the abortion situation in Kenya, Mexico and Poland. Also, researchers need to disseminate better their findings. Those seeking to broaden access to abortion services stand to benefit most, not least because research can undermine prevailing notions of what society thinks it believes about abortion. In all three countries, however, researchers display reservations about working on an issue many fear may prejudice their careers. Moreover, abortion is an extremely personal topic, made even more difficult to study and to discuss because it is illegal in most cases. Inevitably research has not influenced abortion debate as much as in other fields, such as family planning. As one observer told the author, however, the cumulative impact of research findings over time may be likened to waves reaching a beach and beating it into shape.

REFLECTIONS ON THE ABORTION DEBATE

Structures of the debate

In both Kenya and Mexico abortion can be discussed within the cultural realm, and the problem is increasingly recognized as a social reality. However, it is neither fully addressed, nor allowed to enter fully the public sphere. The Kenyan debate underlines several themes common to most African discussions of abortion. These include the lack of clear conceptual categories of debate; the conflict between tradition and modernity, as it pertains to the family; and the reticence of nearly all actors and elites to speak clearly in public about this issue. Thus Kenyans know that abortion is a problem but, as with adolescent fertility and unwanted pregnancy in general, do not know how to talk about a subject surrounded by so much confusion.

The abortion debate in Mexico differs from that in the USA by being more episodic and less public. Abortion has featured intermittently on the public agenda. Positions on abortion are generally more clear-cut than in Kenya, but Mexican governments have been equivocal over the issue. Neither the ruling party nor left-wing groups have mentioned abortion since concerted Church-based pressure brought about the suspension of the 1991 initiative in the state of Chiapas. The debate over abortion engages fewer people and has been less disruptive of the political process than in either Poland or the USA, but it can be no less vitriolic. Abortion has likewise been linked to other points of controversy, especially the role of women in society, making it more complex and difficult to resolve.

In postcommunist Poland debate about abortion has been pervasive at all levels of society and polity. Little of this energy has been channelled into improving education about, and the availability of, more effective contraceptives. The Church initially dominated the debate but could not readily dictate events. Groups were formed to support and oppose the new legal proposals. They organized letter campaigns, petitions and street demonstrations. The use of crusader imagery, anti-clerical demagoguery, the inflexibility of entrenched attitudes and the politicization of the issue produced considerable controversy, shock and fear. The excessive use of rhetorical strategies further prevented a reasoned debate. Not only is the abortion issue subject to conflicting views but the contrasting rubrics that permeated thoughts and actions in the communist period vividly resurfaced in the abortion debate, rendering other categories and attempts at dialogue meaningless. In such circumstances a compromise was most unlikely. The debate reflected the difficulties faced in rebuilding the public sphere as a space for discussing and resolving problems and issues.

Abortion debates are often bitter, divisive and can even be unproductive. In Poland contrasting monologues clashed at the expense of dialogue. Debate has become as polarized and entrenched as in the USA where, since the early 1970s, movement–countermovement interaction has kept two opposing factions constantly mobilized in a conflict that matters far less to an ambivalent majority.[3] Indeed, in both countries, larger and more broadly based constituencies are almost totally absent from the debate. In Poland the Catholic Church and its political allies stress philosophical and moral aspects of abortion, buttressed by nationalistic arguments, whereas groups opposing restrictions on abortion focus on pragmatic and material concerns. In effect, the various contesting parties talk at different levels. A genuine debate is impossible without greater civility and respect for factual accuracy and different beliefs.

In Kenya, Mexico and Poland the dominant discursive frame for abortion is heavily moralistic, overshadowing other concerns. Similarly, one hears the excessively optimistic argument that providing everyone with access to contraceptive information and services will necessarily lead to their adoption. A comparison can be drawn with the failure of many people to practise 'safe sex' in the age of AIDS. Discussing abortion on one plane – as most participants in this debate do – is a gross simplification of a complex issue.

In the USA debate is centred on the notion of competing rights between the pregnant woman and the developing foetus. This arguably makes the search for common ground more difficult and may help explain why the abortion debate has seemingly reached a stalemate.[4] A broader societal compromise has emerged across much of Western Europe where statutes on abortion eschew rights-based rhetoric and disapprove of abortion. Such services are less widely used even though they are readily available in the early stages of pregnancy. In Mexico the concern with rights is more latent than in the USA even if it is the apparent position of feminist groups and many individuals. As in Kenya, human rights are neither well respected nor understood at the individual level. Regardless, the promotion of a 'women's rights' case for abortion is unlikely to receive more support until women assume more power. In Kenya, Mexico and Poland it is difficult to speak of a notion of 'abortion rights', a finding common to many societies. In neo-Confucian cultures, for example, debate about abortion is structured more along collectivist lines, particularly the needs of the society and the family, and the duties owed to them. This has helped enable an authoritarian state such as China, accused of carrying out coercive abortions, to more easily suppress conflict between the state and individuals.

A distinct feature of the abortion debate is the significance of semantics. All players recognize the power of language as an important moulder of concepts and ideas. In Poland especially a number of rhetorical devices have been used for emotional and persuasive effect. By far the most bitter disagreement before and during the 1994 Cairo Conference on Population and Development emerged over the wording of a single paragraph dealing with abortion from the 113-page draft plan of action. The Holy See led efforts to soften, if not eliminate, language intended to urge governments to deal with unsafe abortion. The Church, which speaks of moral norms, would not accept any statement suggesting that abortion could be legal. By contrast, the language of international family planning and development agencies stresses problem-solving and policy options.

It is informed by the empiricism of health and demographic studies. Feminist discourse claims to speak for the marginalized voice of women, thereby emphasizing a third perspective.

Underlying meanings to the debate

It is likely that the basic points of contention regarding abortion have changed little over time. They revolve around questions such as when does life begin? When does the foetus become a person? In what cases may abortion be justified, if at all? Who decides? What role should the state play in formulating policy, and what should be appropriate policy? These problems are perennial. However, the answers given to these questions vary across societies and cultures, depending on prevailing philosophies and institutional structures. Indeed, what is most at stake in the abortion debate varies across countries. There is no country in Western Europe or North America where the abortion debate does not have its own hybrid nature.

On the surface, the abortion debate is about the fate of the foetus. In Kenya, Mexico and Poland the abortion debate is equally a referendum on the appropriate role of women and motherhood in society. This echoes debate in affluent countries where the meaning of abortion varies for women in different social positions and according to their interpretation of the underappreciation of feminine values, especially that of nurturance.[5] Many women in North America and Western Europe came to see legal elective abortion as a symbolic battlecry for their self-determination and equality with men. Other women have opposed abortion to symbolically reaffirm the cultural worth of motherhood and family life in preference to that of the public workplace. But although gender issues are central to abortion debates, gender itself is constructed in different ways across cultures. In Poland, where access to professional occupations has long been open to them, very few women identify with feminism. At the same time, women remain divided over the legal acceptability of abortion. In Mexico and especially in Kenya there are limited opportunities for women seeking alternative avenues of self-development. Demands for a more extensive revision of gender roles have not crystallized in the shape of a broad-based consciousness in favour of 'abortion rights'.

The abortion debate is not only rich in symbolism for many women and women's groups. In Kenya, Mexico and Poland many men and women find troubling any threats to existing societal arrangements, either because they fear change in general, or because they fear the possible effects of increased options for women. This helps explain the irony that those opposed to legalizing abortion tend to oppose efforts to expand access to reliable contraceptives, the most effective means to reduce the incidence of abortion and a major cultural invention of the twentieth century, particularly for women.

Abortion is also a fault line in the ideological politics of the Catholic Church, whose leaders have found internal organizational uses for the abortion issue. In all three countries, particularly Poland and Mexico, the abortion debate is illustrative of church–state tensions and of differences in the social programmes of the Church and liberalism, as is reviewed in the next section. Additionally, debate about abortion reflects a conflict over who runs society. To most secular liberals, the issue boils down to whether one religious group has the right to impose its interpretation of truth on the rest of society. To social conservatives, abortion is often a codeword for the errors of a self-centred liberalism and brings up fears of rampant sex among the young. This conflict has been played out on an epic scale in Poland, where many Catholic bishops continue to see the abortion debate as a battle for the governance of the soul. Many senior Polish bishops have forcefully advocated legal restrictions, thereby giving rise to wider questions of Church-state relations and of the role played by the Church in public life. The debate has further reflected a bitter contest between traditionalists stressing a 'Polish' solution, and liberalists wanting institutions more similar to those of 'the European community of nations'. By invoking such rationalized myths, the abortion debate serves as a forum for a broader struggle over the future shape of society.

Debate about abortion is often reduced to the question of legality, not least because abortion can be defined as a one-dimensional issue judged in terms of who decides whether or not a woman can have an abortion. Moreover, laws can embody and bolster certain definitions and meaning systems over others. They can intensify the abortion debate, particularly if a statute imposes one set of values without attempting to accommodate others. Whereas some researchers have categorized abortion policymaking as 'social regulatory' for seeking to modify human behaviour through public policy,[6] this study suggests that many abortion laws are essentially symbolic in nature and purposefully vague. They represent ideals rather than real commitments. For example, one analyst refers to the

Mexican law as 'a mask of good conscience'.[7] Few Mexicans seem perturbed by this social and ethical contradiction between the imagined reality in the public world and what may happen beyond purview in the private world.

Many Polish churchmen and conservative politicians have insisted that the law can shape morality and behaviour on abortion. Laws can affect social control, but they are not particularly effective in regulating abortion, as illustrated by the failure of the harsh restrictions and penalties imposed by the Ceaușescu regime in Romania. The legal system is equally unable to resolve scientific, ethical or philosophical disputes, such as when life begins or the definition of personhood. There is no consensus in medicine, philosophy or theology on these matters, so it is unrealistic to expect the judiciary to speculate as to the answer.

The abortion debate has served as a mobilizing tool for feminists, traditionalists and the Catholic Church. For example, the Mexican Church has managed to mobilize its faithful at all five phases of debate since the early 1970s, increasing its political profile in the process. In Poland many left-wing politicians continue to treat the issue as a pawn in a political struggle with the Church. Churchmen still equate the legalization of abortion with former communists and with the demands of feminists. The bishops have pressured Catholic politicians over this issue, as has been the case in many countries. Mexican bishops went even further when they excommunicated legislators who passed a liberal abortion law in the state of Chiapas.

The meaning of abortion varies for different groups, giving rise to a number of possible solutions to this debate. Moreover, its meaning changes over time because it is subject to renegotiation.[8] In 1989 the powerful Polish Church and its political allies took the opportunity of systemic change to undermine the provision of abortion and family planning services. The Church sought to redefine a liberal abortion norm by taking advantage of its moral and political strength amidst an institutional vacuum, a search for a new societal order, and a major reassessment of past solutions and all laws inherited from a discredited regime. It attempted to restrict the question of abortion to the scrutiny of Catholic ethics, as defined by the hierarchy.

THE ROLE OF THE CATHOLIC CHURCH IN THE ABORTION DEBATE

More than any other branch of Christianity, the Catholic Church has steadfastly opposed abortion, an issue of undoubted moral and religious concern. Its doctrinal position is clear and has been strongly reiterated by Pope John Paul II. In illuminating the role of the Catholic Church in several different policymaking systems, this study bears out that the level of social and political influence of the Catholic Church is an important determinant of abortion policy.

This influence is qualified by many variables, such as the ideology and power of the ruling regime and the relationship the Church has had with society. However, the Church can be a powerful national grassroots organization even where its activities are restricted. In Kenya the Church has played an important role in nation-building and is deeply concerned with the course of development, though the Church's recent roots and religious competition further make it difficult for Catholic bishops to dominate abortion debate. In Mexico, despite an anti-clerical tradition and constitutional barriers, the Church's case has benefited from the deep cultural roots of Catholic values. It permeates social values even if fewer people practise their faith.[9] The Polish Church in particular is not only a source of faith and moral values. As in Ireland and the Philippines, it is an integral part of the national identity and a critical socio-political operator. In all these countries, the Church has developed the organizational capacity to challenge state policies when it sees fit to do so, such as to prevent attempts to legalize abortion.

Church–state relations and the abortion issue

The Church will always speak out on moral and social issues, but the abortion debate raises age-old questions about the reasonable limits of the Church's involvement (or that of other religious bodies) in the public sphere. It highlights the difficulties of remaining faithful to an ethical position while attempting to develop a public policy that is legislatively feasible. In Catholic countries it also brings up the vexing question of whether the law should mirror the Church's social teachings, as in Ireland or Poland (1993–96), or less directly reflect them, as in Belgium, France, Spain, Portugal or Italy.

These problems are particularly acute in a pluralist society, where public policy must be based on a reasonable consensus within the community, both to achieve its goals and to ensure social peace. Like any other group, the Church can promote its viewpoint and influence the standards of public morality through democratic and non-aggressive means of persuasion.[10] Indeed, this can strengthen the foundations of liberal democracies rather than weaken them as many secularists suggest. At the start of the postcommunist era, however, many within the Polish Church thought they could not talk about abortion as a moral wrong without the institution of a punishment. From an ethical viewpoint, this is not strictly necessary.[11] Many bishops forgot that presenting a moral case against abortion is not the same as making a legal argument against it, a confusion frequently borne out in interviews held with the author. While such tensions exist in many countries, Poland's hierarchy differed in being dominated by those who believed that the Church should organize several areas of public life. By contrast, a 'firm wall' between church and state in the USA has not prevented the Catholic Church developing from a small and insecure base to the largest religious denomination, capable of exerting considerable influence in the public arena. The constitutional separation of church and state has also preserved religious liberty and prevented religious strife, although church–state boundaries remain blurred to some degree.[12] Nevertheless, abortion remains the most sensitive issue in the Catholic relationship with the political arena, one where conservative Catholics and evangelical Protestants have attempted to mould the state to their view.

Although not always accepted, the separation of church and state has been firmly established in Mexico for decades, unlike elsewhere in Latin America. As in Poland, the Church was set in opposition to the state which occasionally disturbed the complex *modus vivendi* that took place at many hidden levels. The policy leverage of the Mexican Church may grow under the new entente with the state that has made Church opposition to abortion legal. On the other hand, this has been *de facto* legitimized for some time. The hierarchy fears that, should it become more assertive, this may provoke resentment and a backlash, given the legacy of church–state and church–society relations. Compared to its Kenyan and Polish counterparts, the Mexican Church has been muted in its criticism of political misrule and has yet to become more active on many social issues.

While the status of church–state relations at any one time sets broad limits on Church engagement in abortion debate, this study has also underscored the indirect political influence which the Church exercises through trusted lay groups which aim to realize its social teachings.[13] These linkages enable a number of penetrative processes. Pro-Vida has increased the Mexican Church's ability to mobilize doctrinally loyal Catholics and its public presence. As in Poland, many devout and militant Catholics have vigorously contested efforts to institute sex education, family planning and AIDS prevention programmes, as well as attempts to legalize abortion. The Church has also exercised influence through Opus Dei which has gained ground in Mexico since the early 1970s, as throughout Latin America.

In Kenya and Mexico governments would rather avoid conflict with the Church over abortion. The state has generally confronted opposition to family planning, but has remained silent over abortion. The Kenyan state is wary of the influence of the Church which, in turn, is respectful of the state's power. In Central America, states are more politically conservative, societies tend to be less anti-clerical, and experience with modern family planning is more recent than in Mexico. This has allowed the Catholic Church there to link abortion more closely to family planning and to attack both more openly and effectively. No Polish government can afford to ignore the Church on an issue it has made so central to national life. After winning a large parliamentary majority in 1993, it took leftist politicians several years before they could successfully confront the Church over the matter, an action that later galvanized opposition against them.

Elsewhere, successive Irish governments have held back from providing contraceptive services. In the Philippines, Asia's largest Christian nation, vocal opposition from Catholic bishops could not resist the expansion of family planning services after the country's first Protestant president assumed office in 1992. Nevertheless, few people are willing to defy the Church more directly, so that, despite growing public health concerns, the state is not prepared to alter abortion policy.[14] In another overwhelmingly Catholic nation, Peruvian President Alberto Fujimori, the Catholic son of Japanese Buddhist immigrants, began his second term in 1995 by calling for free contraceptive distribution as part of a strategy to reduce poverty, but offered few other policies to reduce sharp socio-economic differentials exacerbated by strong market-oriented economic policies.

The Church's position on abortion

The institutional Church has developed a number of sophisticated arguments against abortion. It has often confused the issue, however, as have many who have taken part in abortion debates. In Kenya, Mexico and Poland the author's interviews show that Church leaders still link the cause of abortion law reform to concern about 'overpopulation' which, like the provision of family planning services, need not be connected to neo-Malthusianism.[15] Women, including those from pious Catholic families, in times of crisis do not terminate their pregnancies because they want to, but rather because they feel they cannot bring them to term for a variety of reasons. This condition can be ameliorated through such means as improving contraceptive options. The Church's failure to recognize this fact has mitigated the strength of its defence of the unborn.

In Kenya, Mexico and Poland the implications of religious teachings are strongest for women. Religion is primarily seen as a woman's sphere. It buttresses socio-cultural structures which stress motherhood. The discourse of bishops on abortion deprives women of moral agency by not allowing them to reject what the bishops see as a natural life process. The consequences of such teaching are much greater in poor countries with limited health care services, as throughout much of sub-Saharan Africa. These costs are ignored by the Church's official diagnosis which views abortion above all as a sin. At the same time, churchmen (like politicians and much of society) in Kenya, Mexico, and in many countries, seem content to overlook abortion so long as it is discretely performed and nobody brings up the matter.

In seeking to make abortion a binding moral concern for all Catholics, the rest of the Church's social teaching is downplayed both in the Church's priority of concerns and in the eyes of politicians and the public. In the USA this has prevented the Catholic Church (the largest private health care provider in the country) from lending its considerable weight to supporting the cause of universal health care coverage, a long cherished goal. At the 1994 Cairo Conference on Population and Development, this single-minded focus absorbed a great deal of time and prevented the Church from exercising stronger leadership in projecting the concerns of many economically developing countries, particularly in overcoming the structural inequities between rich and poor nations. And in reasserting the values of homemaking and motherhood, the Church has seemed harshly conservative and hostile to the need for greater gender equality. This perception has reduced the strength of its response to the abortion issue, particularly in more secularized and economically developed nations. It is also at odds with the strong leadership role given by the Catholic Church to the promotion of education and greater respect for women in Kenya and numerous other countries.

Some changes in Church thinking have taken place. Church-based groups have extended aid to unmarried pregnant women. In Poland the Church has engaged more extensively in teaching modern methods of natural family planning than perhaps in any other country. These are promoted as healthy, moral and ecological, although their efficacy is exaggerated and difficulties in using such methods are downplayed or overlooked. Although such changes as occur tend to be evolutionary, the Church does, nonetheless, adapt its structures and teaching over time to cultural, social and other pressures.[16] Its teaching may become more tolerant of contraceptives. Several months before the Cairo conference, the Pontifical Academy of Sciences (a lay body comprising over 80 scientists, some non-Catholic) indirectly advised such a reconsideration, much to the annoyance of the Pope who appoints its members.[17] At Cairo, Church diplomats softened their objections to contraception. Catholics all over the world disregard the papal ban on 'artificial' contraception which they find impractical and which is ineffectual in global terms because it is so widely ignored. Many bishops realize this has damaged episcopal credibility and moral authority and may have weakened their case against abortion. Many also understand the moral inconsistencies of opposing condoms if they can prevent the spread of AIDS.[18] The Church may even develop a more nuanced position regarding abortion, on which its official position has undergone revision in the past.

On the other hand, the Church's principled opposition to abortion has not wavered. John Paul II is leaving behind a formidable moral and doctrinal bequest that will prove difficult to change should his successor want to alter it in any way. He has appointed most of the cardinals who will choose that successor and who are generally thought to share his doctrinal conservatism over sexual morality. The Vatican, which thinks in terms of decades, if not in centuries, is reluctant to alter traditional beliefs. Its rigid teaching over abortion (as over other matters of faith and morals) is structurally reinforced by the hierarchical principle of organization. The laity lacks power and ideological influence within the Church, with dissenters constrained by its non-democratic and elite structure.

Rome's stress on morals lends institutional coherence and helps avoid damaging conflict (internally and externally) over more political concerns, on which its teaching is nonbinding and less precise. In stressing conformity on Church dogma over abortion, therefore, the Vatican is acting to reinforce a global Catholic culture and a relatively coherent belief system from which the Church derives worldwide strength. It is also reasserting doctrinal and administrative control over a transnational and hierarchic organization.[19] John Paul II has given high priority to centralizing authority over faith and morals. Kenyan, Mexican and Polish bishops are united in their public opposition to abortion, if not over how best to communicate that message or to translate it into public policy.

Abortion is an issue that has allowed Church leaders to assume a more public role. Polish bishops saw it as a means to reassert their control and to retain an influential voice in the public arena. They were aware that the Church had been weakened by secularization elsewhere on the continent and that it becomes more difficult for bishops to intervene in electoral politics as democratization proceeds.[20] In the USA the Church's public opposition to the legalization of abortion greatly energized its involvement in national public affairs. This enabled the episcopate to extend its appeals for dignity and respect for human life to include criticisms of economic injustices and national defence policies.[21] Although in neither country has Catholicism persuaded the wider culture, senior Polish bishops informed the author that they had forced a re-evaluation of abortion and an end to its carefree acceptance. Church leaders in Western Europe, however, have been unable to use the abortion debate to create a wedge that would allow them to push other aspects of their public agenda.

The abortion debate is symbolic of several tensions within the worldwide religious body. The hierarchy sees attempts to liberalize abortion as an attack on its teaching about sexual morality and family life. At the same time, its refusal to allow discussion on the matter sits uneasily with the post-Vatican II approach to the modern world and highlights differences of opinion within the Church.[22] The abortion issue has also provided a means for Church leaders to accommodate those still wary of the reforms brought on by the Second Vatican Council, which encouraged a rethinking of almost all aspects of organized Catholicism. However, it has increased rifts over the position of women within that institution and the lack of a deeper gender analysis within its social teaching. Feminist ideas are increasingly filtering into theological debates within the Church. Such voices are pointing out that abortion can be a 'moral' choice, and have criticized the authority of elderly celibate men to decide what is right for women.[23] Rome's patriarchal view of morality will inevitably bring more criticism. It does not have to change its position; but should it not evolve, Rome may also lose an opportunity to take a growing leadership role in the new global culture. Perhaps sensing this, the Vatican appointed a respected legal scholar to head its delegation to the 1995 Fourth UN Conference on Women, the first time it had appointed a woman to lead an official delegation to such a major forum.

In Kenya, Mexico and Poland Catholics resort to abortion quite often because, like non-Catholics, they tend to adopt a more pragmatic approach to life when faced with real-world problems such as an unwanted pregnancy. This is well known to the Church hierarchy, is apparent throughout the Christian world, and finds its complement in societies dominated by such religions as Islam or Hinduism. In this sense, too, lay Catholics are continuing their rejection of the Church's teachings on sexual morality, a trend highlighted by the controversy over *Humanae Vitae*. The matter is of great concern to John Paul II whose tenth encyclical, *Veritatis Splendor* ('The splendor of truth'), implored bishops to stress the moral content of faith.[24]

OBSTACLES TO INSTITUTING MORE LIBERAL ABORTION POLICIES

This study indicates that the opposition of the Catholic Church and dominant public ideas concerning the role of women, who lack decision-making power, pose major barriers to the adoption of more liberal abortion policies. The lack of reliable data and the low priority of women's health concerns makes it difficult to draw attention to abortion-related problems. In Kenya and Mexico there is an unwillingness to address this issue, which is clouded further by the disruption of sexual and reproductive norms. Policy elites perceive a high degree of risk and uncertainty should they open up debate on abortion. As in Poland, there is a lack of consensus as to what should be appropriate abortion policy. Politicians generally avoid the issue because they find it expedient to say nothing.

Attempts to liberalize abortion policy are often defused by a system of bias that favours the status quo and prevents awkward issues from arising.[25] In 1976, for example, Mexican policy elites considered defining abortion as a health problem for women. An expert commission duly called for the legalization of abortion, but the outgoing government did not take up the recommendations that were abandoned by its successor. Governments have subsequently postponed decision-making and suppressed an unresolved debate after they or other groups had mooted proposals to legalize abortion, most recently in 1991. These varied responses echo the three major strategies of avoidance, postponement and de-politicization that have characterized how Western European governments have sought to deal with such controversy.[26] Although non-public decision-making is difficult to analyse, a policy of inaction is currently preferred. This effectively becomes a decision that favours one side to the debate.

The dearth of political will to review abortion policy also stems from doubts as to the efficacy and morality of legalizing the procedure as a means to reducing its incidence, and the relative ease with which all major parties are relieved of the responsibility of addressing the dilemmas surrounding abortion whenever family planning is offered as a solution. Policymakers are unwilling to take on an issue that offers them little gain, and where they find it difficult to align facts with values and to mediate between the different parties in this dispute.

In Kenya and Mexico there is little manifest public demand or domestic pressure to force a shift in government policy. Indeed, for most people in the poorer regions of the world, and for women in particular, broader aspects of health and survival, as well as caring for young children, are of greater concern than abortion. With systemic change in Poland, urgent economic problems and the new fear of losing one's job inevitably concerned most women more than new restictions placed on abortion. In all three countries, women's health has been identified primarily with maternal health needs which have been addressed chiefly through services oriented towards the child.[27] Many other pressing health concerns, including AIDS, compete for policy attention. Consequently the issue of abortion may have to transcend the health sphere to be seriously considered by policymakers.

Kenya and Mexico are hubs of international agencies and have strong ties with economically developed countries. Governments have implemented population and safe motherhood programmes but are reluctant to move on the issue of abortion because they fear polarization and a potential backlash against their population policies. It may be that rather than risk controversy by changing the law, many Latin American and African governments would prefer to turn a blind eye to the existing situation, let restrictive abortion laws lapse, and permit, but not openly encourage, private initiatives discretely to establish abortion services where feasible. For their part, medical, family planning and other potentially reform-minded groups are reluctant to promote change openly without a signal from the government. As one Mexican family planning leader who favoured legalizing abortion told the author: 'Nobody wants to touch the issue. Nothing will happen despite the efforts of feminists and others unless the President suddenly favors it, at which point, all institutions would just accept orders and do it ... the real public health masters in Mexico are the government employees who receive their instructions.'

The limited effectiveness of reform-minded groups

In Kenya, Mexico and Poland non-governmental actors active on the abortion issue (including anti-abortion groups, but excluding the Catholic Church) remain small and underfunded, and find it difficult to maintain momentum. They lack organizational experience, in large part because associational life has been restricted by the state. There has been no effective grassroots challenge to existing laws in Kenya and Mexico. Even in postcommunist Poland, new NGOs are hampered by limited public confidence and face profound organizational difficulties. Governments are more likely to listen to the Catholic Church which commands greater organizational resources, political skill and legitimacy.

Physicians have generally adopted a low-key profile except for some gynaecologists who have stressed the adverse health consequences of unsafe abortion. Their professional organizations carry none of the political clout held by their counterparts in rich countries. Family planning agencies are still less powerful and evince divided opinions over abortion. For legal, political and funding reasons, they are reluctant to involve themselves in programmes which they perceive might harm them. On the other hand, several population and health agencies have sought to improve post-abortion services and to propagate improved procedures for managing incomplete abortion cases. The Cairo conference further legitimized such work in the eyes of the international community, but, to date, the matter is being given little political attention or financial provision.

In Kenya, Mexico and Poland health specialists, family planners and feminists have failed to develop strategic alliances to reduce abortion incidence and work towards affecting policy changes. Efforts at greater cooperation tend to be undermined by institutional envies and suspicions. Few are talking about setting up para-legal channels to improve abortion services. In the international arena, feminist, health and family planning communities drew more closely together during the early 1990s, particularly in redefining abortion as part of a broader package of concerns over reproductive health, an agenda so far set primarily by Western groups. Women's health advocates, particularly from the United States, lobbied effectively to shape the agenda and programme of the 1994 UN International Conference on Population and Development. This reached a consensus on the need to improve the status of women, as did the 1995 Beijing Conference on Women. However, the first day of the Cairo meeting was marked by strong and conflicting calls both for the acceptance and the rejection of abortion from the female heads of state of Norway and Pakistan, respectively.[28] Women are becoming more adept at drawing attention to issues that concern them, but there are differences in the relative strengths and agendas of women's groups across – and within – countries.

In Kenya, Mexico and Poland women's groups remain relatively powerless and divided. Most lack a clear, goal-oriented programme. They have been neither adept at pooling their resources nor in seeking coalition partners. Entrenched interests collude to render feminist discourse ineffective. This is dismissed as too radical and, like abortion itself, alien to native traditions and harmful to motherhood and national survival. One feminist intellectual in Poland suggested to the author that 'this image problem accounts for 90 percent of the reason why feminism is easily attacked and discredited'. As in Kenya and Mexico, there is a difference between feminist thinking and what most regard as a general but non-feminist involvement with women's issues. A feminist agenda is shared by a few economically well-to-do women who tend to receive help from domestic maids, sisters or aunts and can obtain a safe abortion. Married women find the cause of abortion law reform difficult to support and most suffer the double burden of domestic and salaried work.

Women's groups advocating a more liberal abortion policy find themselves in a strategic quandary. They have often adopted a discourse manufactured in the West and applied it in a setting where feminism is poorly understood. Taken crudely, such strategies all too often pit 'us' against 'them' (men). Moreover, advocates of legal abortion seeking to frame debate as a rights issue are likely to find such a strategy both ineffective and counterproductive where such arguments are not well inculcated and there is insufficient institutional capacity to handle debate on such grounds. In Kenya as for most of Africa, rights are treated as if they are a gift from the rulers to the *wanachi*, or people, whose awareness of legal rights is quite low. Pitching women's rights against foetal rights would dichotomize and confound the question of what to do about abortion. It would also shift debate further towards the moral and ethical planes, enabling traditionalists and the Catholic Church to emphasize their positions more clearly.

The Mexican group GIRE was formed out of ideological and tactical disillusion with past feminist activities. It possesses few resources but has achieved strong initial results through greater cooperation with reform-oriented groups and communicating a new discourse on abortion. This is centred on a greater tolerance for diverse opinions and develops the themes of 'choice' and reproductive rights. It remains to be seen how far these arguments will be accepted, not least because they cannot be isolated from larger socio-economic structures.

LOOKING TO THE FUTURE

It seems probable that the tensions that mark the contemporary abortion debate will continue. Technological innovations have made abortion a safer procedure, but they have neither dispelled controversy, nor are they likely to do so soon. The potential spread of mifepristone and even more effective antiprogestins may blur the distinction between contraception and abortion, and make abortion a more private matter. However, this is unlikely to resolve conflict or transcend it, since mifepristone works only in cases of early pregnancy and access to it is deeply embedded in the larger abortion debate. Other technological developments may also open up controversy in unforeseen ways. For example, amniocentesis and ultrasound machines (two technologies designed for diagnostic purposes and pregnancy monitoring) have been widely misused for sex-selective abortion in a number of South and East Asian countries, distorting sex ratios at young age groups.[29]

The future course of the abortion debate will also vary across states according to the influences of the USA and Rome. The abortion issue is likely to remain high on the public agenda within the USA, from where advocacy groups of diverse persuasions are increasingly reaching out to influence abortion policies in other countries. US government policies on abortion may again be substantially altered by presidential and electoral changes, with significant international implications. A future pope and his preferred advisers may give less emphasis to abortion, while bishops may prefer to stress other concerns. However, the Vatican is unlikely to modify its teaching on abortion, which will remain a delicate matter in church–state relations. In Poland and Mexico these have entered a new phase and it is unclear what forms of mutual accommodation will result, and with what consequences for the way abortion is considered.

The contours of the abortion debate continue to evolve, and merit close observation in all three countries examined in detail here. Kenya is a country still looked at for providing clues to future developments in Africa, even though it is no longer one of the continent's more open societies. Mexico commands similar attention in Latin America. Any revisions of abortion policy in these countries could have a demonstration effect elsewhere in their regions. While controversy over abortion will probably grow in both Mexico and Kenya, the dispute in Poland is now as overdichotomized and polemical as in the USA. Its tone and frames of reference are set by advocates who talk at different levels and about different things, using emotionally charged rhetoric, often for their own political and social gain. A more informed debate requires greater tolerance from all sides and a realization that the reality of abortion for a woman has little to do with such rhetoric. In the meantime, the implications of public health data are clear, particularly with regard to the complications of poorly performed procedures. A greater focus on the incidence of abortion, with public policy directed to that end, would help decrease the scale of existing problems. All participants in this debate agree that abortion is best avoided, though not necessarily that policies oriented towards preventing unwanted pregnancies are the best solution.

There may be no answer to the policy conundrum posed by abortion that will satisfy all belligerents. This does not preclude some sort of working compromise. Indeed, a number of societies have reached such a position. This is disturbing for an issue that concerns the essence of life itself. However, it is preferable to an un-remitting and bitter struggle over a topic that has many moral ambiguities. Such a judgement does not absolve society from continuing to search for a situation where divergent views may be at least better accommodated, if not wholly reconciled. The question of what to do about abortion will remain controversial; but, like any other problem, it should always be debatable.

Appendix

The research presented in this book is based on multiple sources of evidence. The use of three data-collection strategies strengthened its validity, ironing out inconsistencies, minimizing uncertainties and deepening understanding. First, I maintained a field diary to record my observations and reflections, the literature I read, and whom I met and interviewed. Second, I conducted a series of open-ended, semi-structured interviews with key officials, activists and informed observers in each country. I also held discussions with officials of various sub-national, national and international agencies based in the USA, London and elsewhere. Third, I examined a wide range of written sources including official documents, academic articles, newspaper accounts, the literature and statements of professional and interest groups, as well as survey data on contraceptive use and estimates of abortion.

I sought to engage myself deeply in each country to become familiar with the way things are. This permitted understanding the way abortion is considered both from the viewpoint of an insider with a developed sensitivity to local conditions, as well as from the perspective of someone outside that setting, conversant with the issues involved and holding the analytical distance required of a scholar. This enabled the results of the study to be firmly grounded empirically and conceptually.

The approach resembles what has been called 'grounded theory', an inductive strategy for generating and confirming theory stemming from close involvement with real-world patterns.[1] In seeking to make this study more participatory and holistic, I have also been informed by elements of ethnographic research, which seeks to understand what people are thinking in terms of cultural and linguistic meanings;[2] by more recent explorations of discourse theory and communicative action, which examine variations within the discourses of groups that stake claims to validity and to defining aspects of everyday life;[3] and by reflecting more directly on what I experienced among those involved or interested in this drama.[4] The policymaking process itself is primarily observed and explained through the use of elite theory and models of policymaking, as explained in Chapter 1. Therefore, the research findings are additionally interpreted from a political, and not just a social or cultural perspective.

The research process had clear chronological sequence, although different stages intermixed and overlapped. Data collection commenced at least one year prior to fieldwork in each country and included literature searches, building up a list of likely contacts and people worth interviewing, and tapping into existing networks of organizations and information. However, the great bulk of material was only available in Kenya, Mexico and Poland. Fieldwork began in Kenya, late 1991, and continued for about a year with short breaks in between the trips. In all three countries, the fieldwork was mostly conducted in the capital city, the site of the greatest

173

concentration of resources and where the larger part of influence- and decision-making takes place. Field trips beyond the capital cities were made as appropriate, particularly to comprehend critical cases better (such as the southern Mexican state of Chiapas) and local variations in the treatment of the issue. Follow-up trips were made to Mexico and Poland in 1993 and 1994, and information continued to be gathered in all three countries thereafter.

To the extent that it is possible to do so, I used an amalgam of methods to gauge as closely as possible the approximate incidence of abortion and its fertility-inhibiting effects. This included evaluating official statistics (available only for Poland, where they are incomplete) and hospital admissions data, community-based and other survey data (on abortion incidence or contraceptive practice), and developing an understanding of the 'illegal abortion system' by garnering locally available evidence, such as through talking with health care staff and those knowledgeable about the situation. The application of the proximate determinants framework for analysing fertility patterns offers another indirect technique for estimating the scale and demographic impact of abortion. It yields indices for the intermediate variables (such as contraceptive use and marital patterns, as well as abortion) that directly affect fertility, ranging in value from 0.0 (which implies zero fertility) to 1.0 (implying no effect on fertility).[5] However, the utility of all these estimation approaches is heavily qualified by the weak quality of existing data. Indeed, abortion statistics tend to be reliable only where abortion is accepted and sanctioned, abortion services are sufficient and adequate, most abortions are performed in registered institutions, and there is good compliance with reporting procedures. Survey data and questionnaire research tend to substantially underreport induced abortion, even where its practice is legal.[6]

All three countries posed difficult environments for conducting research on a phenomenon that remains unlawful and stigmatized in nearly all cases. On some occasions, the author came across individuals suspicious of his work, asking many questions as to its purpose and funding. By comparison, it is now much easier to investigate issues concerned with contraception in Kenya and Mexico. In these countries the institutional base provided by Pathfinder International (a family planning agency) facilitated my access to the health care and research communities. In Kenya this help came at a time when many people were afraid to talk about any controversial issue, particularly if their comments might in any way be construed as implicating the government. This made access to information problematic, not least to understanding the opaque inner dynamics of the policymaking process.

I conducted most of my fieldwork in Poland during a time of breathtaking change. This made all aspects of life difficult to describe and to follow, and the research process even more exciting and challenging. It further coincided with a rapid rise in scepticism about the worth of many poorly informed 'Western' consultants and survey researchers who began to work in the region. In addition, much of the fieldwork took place when the abortion debate was particularly intense and continuously unfolding. One meeting with an adjunct minister was abruptly interrupted when the interviewee was summoned to be dismissed from office for holding different views from those favoured by the current government.

Although all data sources were treated as complementary to each other so as to prevent any facts or perceptions from being overemphasized or misstated, the interviews proved to be the primary research tool. A total of 162 interviews were conducted, counting only situations that lasted for over one hour of solid interviewing; anything shorter was considered a discussion or a conversation. The interviews yielded much information unavailable by other means, along with many useful perspectives and reflections on the issues and questions under study. They also enabled the author to develop further his own ideas about the data.

The sampling involved both purposeful and snowball procedures. Accordingly, on the basis of my readings, discussions and other enquiries, I selected organizations and individuals known to be active in the abortion debate; those exercising authority and influence on deliberations about abortion policy and those close to them; and those cognizant of this and related aspects of the abortion situation relevant to the study. I also looked for key informants mentioned by interviewees, who often gave me referrals and sometimes arranged the contact themselves. Most of the interviews were set up following telephone calls and then held in people's homes or offices. Elite and sub-elite organizational leaders were drawn from different organizational categories. They included high-level officials and their advisers; leading figures from domestic and international groups with stakes in the policymaking process; academics and researchers; key members of associations or professional groups such as physicians (particularly obstetricians) and family planning personnel; feminists, civil libertarians and other activists; journalists and various knowledgeable individuals and qualified informants.[7]

A number of open-ended questions were asked to elicit information on how different actors defined particular problems, situations or processes. Questions were framed in such a way as to provide points of comparison between different interviews *per se* and between the three countries. Often, the evidence obtained was suggestive rather than definitive. However, this is usually the case in such research, reinforcing the need to confirm findings through additional sources of information. Attempts were made to interview informants from a group or institution separately, so as to guard against the chance of distorted data or interpretation, and to increase familiarity with a particular organization. I kept several perceptive analysts and interviewees informed of my work so as to solicit feedback and check on the veracity and progress of my research.

The interviews lasted on average two hours, excluding breaks or peripheral conversation. I often tried to obtain a second interview with those particularly informative, articulate, and who could seemingly shed light on matters that eluded me. This allowed me to think more about follow-up questions, to pursue other leads, and to read over materials lent to me. Also, the interviewee was invariably more relaxed as to the nature of my enquiry. All meetings were conducted very carefully because of the moral, cultural and political overtones to the issues concerned. Many of the identities of my informants have been kept secret in the text to protect their confidentiality where necessary, and to respect requests for anonymity. Catholic bishops, for example, must show loyalty to the official teachings of their institution, with senior bishops appointed for their obedience, among other qualities. Hence their names have not been cited if they revealed information that could harm their interests. Interviewing physicians likewise required particular discretion in all three countries.

The Kenyan study is based on 46 interviews (42 conducted in Kenya, four more in the USA) and nine follow-up interviews. Two interviews lasted over seven hours, excluding breaks, and some extended over the course of several days. The Kenyan work consists, therefore, of a minimum of 55 interviews. For Mexico, I carried out 50 interviews, two being held in the USA, and 12 of which were follow-up interviews. In Poland, I interviewed 45 people, ten of whom granted second interviews, and I conducted two more interviews in the USA and London. The interviews were recorded in shorthand, with the detailed notes transcribed as soon as possible and then reviewed to define subsequent lines of enquiry. I almost never taped interviews, as this seemed off-putting and disruptive.

In addition, I gathered reports from newspapers in Kenya, Mexico and Poland, as well as the United States and Britain, so as to follow the course of abortion debate and to secure the names of people interested in it. Such materials cannot be used uncritically. As is well known, the mass media often oversimplify, if not bypass, facts. Journalists do not usually state their sources of information. Far greater problems of validity are posed by media constraints in non-democratic countries, where journalists may be intimidated from challenging official interpretations of events. On the other hand, elites talk to each other through different sectors of the press, even if these outlets are heavily controlled. In other words, the press is a forum for elite (if not societal) debate, underlining the relevance of such data. Journals and newspapers also illustrate what is judged locally, nationally and internationally as significant in the social world.

Notes

1 A Global Policy Conundrum

1. Unless otherwise noted, abortion is taken to mean 'induced abortion', the deliberate termination of a pregnancy before the foetus is capable of independent life outside the womb. By contrast, a 'spontaneous abortion', or miscarriage, refers to a nonviable foetus, that is to say, any involuntarily induced abortion, even where an external cause such as trauma, accident or disease is involved.

2. The author is well aware that these three countries do not span the globe. The reasons for selecting these countries are specified further at the end of this chapter and at the start of each subsequent chapter. It would have been desirable to conduct fieldwork in additional settings, but limitations of finance, time and energy precluded this possibility.

3. For further discussion see Jung and Shannon (1988); and Byrnes and Segers (1992).

4. See Coleman (1991); and Williams and Houck (1993) for thoughtful reviews. In 1891 Pope Leo XII issued the encyclical *Rerum Novarum* ('Of new things'), which showed great concern for the wretched conditions of workers caught up in the new and often violent process of industrial capitalism then sweeping across Europe. This is often taken to be the start of the Church's modern social doctrine, although such teaching has always been a part of its mission.

5. Here, I refer to 'liberalism' in its classical sense, by which I include capitalism and liberal ideologies such as freedom of religious practice, and the separation of church and state. Elsewhere in this study, I use the term 'liberal' in the modern sense, meaning a centre-left perspective.

6. In many countries, Christianity has played a facilitating role in democratic crafting. In his dealings with politicians and in his teachings, Pope John Paul II has strongly and consistently emphasized the need to respect human dignity and rights. Regarding the movement towards democracy in world politics, see Huntington (1991); and Diamond and Plattner (1993).

7. The Tbilisi Declaration (reprinted in Newman, 1993) further recommended ways to improve the management of abortion and reduce its incidence, particularly through better contraceptive use.

8. See Okagbue (1990) on the Nigerian case which closely reflects the Kenyan situation. Knoppers *et al.* (1990) review how French laws affected statutes governing abortion in Francophone Africa.

9. For example, by 1975, France, Austria and Sweden had adopted the first trimester of pregnancy as the time limit until when a woman and her physician could decide about abortion. This was the same framework employed by the US Supreme Court in its landmark 1973 decision.

The roles played by the Supreme Court and state legislatures in the US abortion debate are described by Judges (1993).

10. The impact of abortion on fertility rates can also be measured indirectly, given good data on trends in contraception, nuptiality and breastfeeding (Bongaarts and Potter, 1983; and Frejka, 1983).

11. For example, sociological profiles of female activists engaged in the US abortion dispute are provided by Luker (1984); and F. Ginsburg (1989). See E.A. Cook *et al.* (1992) for an examination of public attitudes about abortion and some of their ramifications.

12. See, for example, Noonan (1970); and Connery (1977) on the development of Catholic teaching on abortion; and Mussalam (1983) on Islamic teaching about abortion.

13. Comparative legal assessments are provided by Frankowski and Cole (1987); Glendon (1987); and R.J. Cook (1989). See also the three-volume international compendium of abortion laws and policies produced by the United Nations (UN, 1992; 1993; and 1995a).

14. See, for example, Callahan (1970); and Callahan and Callahan (1984).

15. See Devereux (1976) for a detailed tabulation of traits associated with abortion in many former cultures; and Riddle (1992) for a review of the techniques of abortion and contraception mentioned in Western writings from antiquity to the seventeenth century.

16. Koop (1989: 175). The major reasons cited were the use of experimental designs betraying the personal biases of authors, and methodological problems such as denial by respondents that they have had an abortion. President Ronald Reagan appointed C. Everett Koop as the US Surgeon General from 1981 to 1989, in part for his personal opposition to abortion. The Surgeon General declined to write a report on the health and psychological effects of abortion commissioned to help justify restricting abortion services. He found insufficient evidence to justify such a move.

17. In what may be the most thorough study and anthology available, David *et al.* (1988) examined the developmental effects of denied abortion from childhood through adolescence to early adulthood. Although inconclusive, the evidence suggests that 'unwanted' children tend to do less well in school, are more prone to mental health problems and trouble with the law, and are less likely to be satisfied with their lives as adults than 'wanted' children. These findings are confirmed by the fourth wave of data collection from the ongoing 'Prague Study', the methodologically soundest study to date (Kubicka *et al.*, 1995).

18. Broad-ranging discussions of how abortion levels and trends may change over the course of fertility transition, and with what effect on aggregate fertility levels, are offered by Requena-Bichet (1970); and Tietze and Bongaarts (1976). See also Bongaarts (1990) on how levels and trends of wanted and unwanted births vary over the course of the fertility transition.

19. The total fertility rate (TFR) refers to the average number of children a woman would have at the end of her reproductive lifetime if she experienced the currently observed fertility rates (of a given year) throughout her childbearing years. Given a low mortality situation, a

TFR of about 2.1 is regarded as replacement level fertility, sufficient in the long term to maintain population size.

20. Frejka (1983); and Ketting (1993).
21. Viel (1988); and Frejka and Atkin (1996).
22. See Coeytaux (1988); and Rogo (1996)
23. Bongaarts and Potter (1983).
24. This proportion cannot be readily computed. However, spontaneous abortions are thought to occur in about 15 per cent of all pregnancies that survive to clinical recognition (which occurs at around five to seven weeks after the last menstrual period), after which the probability of foetal loss decreases with gestational age (Kline *et al.*, 1989).
25. See Henshaw and Morrow (1990) for comparative statistics on many countries for which reliable data are known; and Popov (1991) for a review of the situation in the former Soviet Union, where rates are especially high in the central region of European Russia.
26. The fall in US abortion rates may be due to an increase in the number of births to unmarried women; greater acceptance of single parenting; a higher proportion of women moving into the older, less fecund end of their childbearing years; more restrictions on access to abortion (Henshaw and van Vort, 1994); and increased contraceptive use among young people.
27. Gynaecologists in particular profit from the high number of abortions performed. Many observers believe this is the major reason why the Japanese medical profession continues to oppose distribution of the contraceptive pill (a method widely used elsewhere, particularly among non-parous women), rather than because of its professed concern for women's health (S. Coleman, 1983).
28. WHO (1992). This definition was adopted as a footnote to paragraph 8.25 (which dealt with abortion) of the Programme of Action adopted by the 1994 Cairo Conference on Population and Development (UN, 1995b).
29. WHO/UNICEF (1996). For earlier estimates, see Royston and Armstrong (1989); and WHO (1994). However, reliable maternal mortality data do not exist for most poor countries (Mauldin, 1994).
30. The WHO recommends vacuum aspiration as the preferred method. Manual vacuum aspiration is leading to improved abortion care and reduced treatment costs for incomplete abortion in many poor countries, including Kenya and Mexico (B.R. Johnson *et al.*, 1992; and Greenslade *et al.*, 1993).
31. For further information about the sequelae of abortion and their consequences, see Grimes (1995). The largest and most comprehensive study to date found no overall increased risk of breast cancer from induced abortion (Melbye *et al.*, 1997).
32. Mifepristone has been identified as a possible treatment for endometriosis, uterine fibroma, Cushing's syndrome (a rare adrenal gland disease), Parkinson's disease and breast cancer. Van Look and von Hertzen (1994) describe the development and operation of mifepristone and other antiprogestins.

33. Crenin and Vittinghoff (1994); and Hausknecht (1995). Larger studies are still needed to ascertain the reliability of this alternative approach to performing abortion in the early stage of pregnancy.
34. As assessed by the Population Division of the United Nations (UN, 1998) and the research unit of the Alan Guttmacher Institute, which monitors abortion trends (Henshaw and Morrow, 1990).
35. For more details see UN (1992; 1993; and 1995a). Chile and Malta, however, neither legally permit abortion under any circumstances, nor have any implicit statute provisions that would lawfully allow abortion where it could save the life of a woman.
36. The Soviet Union legalized abortion on broad grounds in 1920 and again in 1955 after outlawing it in 1936. See R.J. Cook (1989) on the worldwide trend towards liberalization of abortion laws in the 1970s and 1980s.
37. Although stated as dominant concerns, public health considerations were secondary motives for the legalization of abortion in all four countries. Note that, in India, deaths and morbidity remain common due to the limited provision of legal abortion services, particularly in rural areas where most people live (Chhabra and Nuna, 1994). See Oakley (1977: 234–47) on the development of abortion policy in Japan; and Besemeres (1980) regarding the former Soviet Union.
38. Menstrual regulation is usually performed manually using a syringe and a cannula. The procedure is carried out without pregnancy testing and typically within the first two weeks after a missed menstrual period, an event that many cultures differentiate from a confirmed pregnancy. It is often popularly referred to as 'bringing on a late period', or 'bringing it down'.
39. David and Pick de Weiss, 1992; and Paxton *et al.*, 1993.
40. For further details, see Hord *et al.* (1991); and B.R. Johnson *et al.* (1993).
41. Henshaw and van Vort (1994).
42. For more information, see the essays assembled by Lovenduski and Outshoorn (1986).
43. See Inglis (1987) on the 1983 referendum, as well as on the influence of the Catholic Church in Irish public life more generally; and Francome (1992) on the 1992 referendum and the characteristics of the approximately 5,000 Irish women who travel each year to England for abortions. Ireland and England share the same legal system, including many laws; but whereas England legalized abortion in 1967, the procedure remains essentially illegal in Ireland. The 1967 British Abortion Act did not extend to Northern Ireland, a part of the United Kingdom.
44. For a longer discussion see Kingdon (1995), who refers to such moments as 'policy windows'. Other authors (for example, Tarrow, 1994) refer to political opportunity structures, particularly in describing the political conditioning of collective action.
45. The thalidomide tragedy was vividly brought to life for many Americans by the case of Sherry Finkbine, a mother of four children who in 1962 travelled to Sweden to obtain an abortion. having correctly feared she had a thalidomide-deformed foetus. Soon afterwards, the 1964–65

epidemic of rubella led to many more cases of severe birth defects (Luker, 1984).

46. Hereafter, unless otherwise noted, the 'Church' refers to the Catholic Church.
47. Informed discussions of the ways by which this influence may be exerted are provided by Hanson (1987); Reese (1996); and Vallier (1972).
48. During the Second Vatican Council, the world's Catholic bishops gathered in four sessions to re-examine the nature of the Church and its relation to the world. They instituted the most radical Church reforms since the Council of Trent (1546–63), which was held as a response to the Protestant Reformation.
49. At the UN, the Holy See (the office or jurisdiction of the Pope) maintains permanent observer status, entitling it to participate in policy discussions and conferences, but not to vote in the UN's General Assembly.
50. Goldscheider and Mosher (1991); and Sander (1992). However, Greeley (1990) shows that American Catholics have remained in the Church despite the frequent discrepancy between their own beliefs and behaviours and the teachings of the hierarchy, particularly over birth control.
51. In the USA for example, the percentage of women obtaining abortions who profess to be Catholic is comparable to the percentage of Catholics in the general population (Henshaw and Kost, 1996).
52. Extensive scholarly treatments of the development of Catholic doctrine on abortion are offered by Callahan (1970: 409–47); Noonan (1970); and Connery (1977). See also the critiques by Hurst (1989), whose brief survey stresses the changes that have occurred in Church teaching on abortion; and Ranke-Heinemann (1990), whose provocative account sets that teaching in a context of how churchmen have often slighted the concerns of women.
53. Until the development of modern medical technology, a pregnancy could not be confirmed until quickening. Under common law before the nineteenth century, abortion was not considered an offence if performed before quickening and was considered a misdemeanour rather than a felony if performed after quickening.
54. John Paul II (1995).
55. See, for example, Byrnes (1991); and Byrnes and Segers (1992).
56. Opus Dei was set up in 1928 in Spain. The movement is favoured by Pope John Paul II who in 1982 granted it the unique status of a 'personal prelature'. This gives it relative autonomy within the Church hierarchy, permitting it to appoint its own priests and conduct its own affairs. This is one reason why many liberal Catholics think it wields excessive influence and accuse it of being a cult within the Church (Walsh, 1989; and Lernoux, 1989).
57. For more information about this group, see Byrnes and Segers (1992: 169–84). Many theologians and bishops have also recognized the difficulty in squaring Vatican teaching on contraception and abortion, although bishops are most unlikely to voice disagreement with the *magisterium* publicly.

58. For example, Donaldson (1990: 9–17) cites instances from the 1970s of strong opposition to government-backed contraceptive services from some senior American prelates. Their efforts were not equally shared by most Catholics and proved less of an obstacle to international family planning assistance than commonly believed.
59. As listed in article II, section 12, of the 1987 constitution. For an account of Church and other influences on population, family planning and reproductive health issues in the Philippines, see Desiderio (1993).
60. The 800-page 'Catechism of the Catholic Church' is a compendium of Church teachings intended to guide all Catholics. It is the first official manual of doctrine in more than four centuries and, perhaps more significantly, since the Second Vatican Council (Holy See, 1994).
61. As underscored by the Pope's major encyclicals on the social concerns of the Church, *Sollicitudo rei socialis* (John Paul II, 1988) and *Centesimus annus* (John Paul II, 1991).
62. John Paul II (1981). The book was first published in Poland two decades earlier. In his biography of John Paul II, Szulc (1995) also pointed to the likely connections between Wojtyła's book and Pope Paul VI's encyclical.
63. Paul VI (1968: paragraph 14). The encyclical reaffirmed that Catholic married couples should not use any form of birth control other than abstinence or the rhythm method, which Pope Pius XII sanctioned in 1951. There is a large literature on the controversy surrounding the encyclical. See, for example, Seidler and Meyer (1989: 92–108); Keely (1994); and McClory (1995).
64. Indeed, American and British physicians had first captured this professional area of autonomy in the nineteenth century (Mohr, 1978; Imber, 1986; and Keown, 1988). See also Petersen (1993) on the Australian case. Note that the views of physicians and organized medical groups have changed over time, chiefly for reasons of professional self-interest.
65. See McKeegan (1992); and Petchesky (1990: 241–85) on the New Right movement, which lost momentum by the early 1990s. A comprehensive scholarly study of the 'pro-life' movement in the USA is still lacking, however.
66. The violent nature of confrontation over abortion in the USA is investigated by Blanchard and Prewitt (1993). Their study focuses on Pensacola, a small town in Florida that became a magnet for militants on both sides of the abortion debate well before two physicians providing abortion services and a security escort were murdered there in 1993 and 1994.
67. Donaldson (1990: 49–51) notes that, in the 1970s, US government contributions made up about 40 per cent or more of all international population assistance, or close to 50 per cent if one added private funds. The USA continues to be the largest population donor in aggregate terms.
68. The Reagan administration's first Ambassador to the Holy See, with which the USA established formal diplomatic relations in 1984, later

attested to Vatican influence in the formation of the 'Mexico City policy' ('The U.S. and the Vatican on birth control', *Time*, 24 February 1992, p. 35).

69. See Fox (1986) on how the policy came into being; Camp (1987) on its adverse impacts for women and children; and Blane and Friedman (1990) on its implementation within family planning programmes worldwide. The 'promotion' of abortion was later defined to include counselling, referral and non-pejorative information.

70. Camp and Lasher (1989) describe the record of the Reagan administration's hostility to US international population policy. While ethical violations have been committed in China's family planning programme, there is no evidence that UNFPA has ever contributed to them.

71. 'Clinton orders reversal of abortion restrictions left by Reagan and Bush', *New York Times*, 23 January 1993.

72. The Nairobi conference adopted the 'Forward-looking Strategies for the Advancement of Women'. This document proved a valuable tool in helping women gain greater control over their own lives. See Petchesky and Weiner (1990); and Dixon-Mueller (1993) on the growth of feminist interest in the reproductive health concerns of women in poor countries.

73. Adopted in 1995, the IPPF's Charter on Sexual and Reproductive Rights embodies 12 rights including 'the right to life which means, among other things, that no woman's life should be put at risk or endangered by reason of pregnancy', and 'that all persons must be free to enjoy and control their sexual and reproductive life' (IPPF, 1996a).

74. Crane (1994) outlines how transnational groups (particularly 'pro-choice' groups) have become active on the world scene, seen through the prism of groups operating in the USA.

75. 'Russians and Americans join in anti-abortion fight', *New York Times*, 19 May 1994. During one of his interviews, the author was unexpectedly invited to assist several prominent North American anti-abortion activists due to visit Poland and Lithuania.

76. Human Life International's activities in Zambia have included strong support for the Family Life Movement of Zambia, which has also attempted to alter sex education programmes in schools (Cremins, 1984); and the financing of a 'pro-life' conference in 1989 which attracted several hundred people from twelve countries, of which six were African (Human Life International Newsletter, Special Report no. 61, November 1989).

77. In South Korea, abortion became widely practised during the 1960s and legalized in 1973, by when the number of abortions exceeded that of births in Seoul. The legal change was opposed by the small Catholic minority and some Protestant groups (Potts *et al.*, 1977).

78. D. Callahan (1970: 155–6) points out that the very small Catholic minority in India presented more opposition to the legalization of abortion than did the Hindu majority. See LaFleur (1992) on the ways in which Japanese society (which is made up of neo-Shintoist, neo-Confucianist, and Buddhist influences) copes with the conflicting emotions associated with a high abortion rate. For a comparative survey

of how the world's major religions have treated abortion, see Kulczycki (1997).

79. There is a consensus among all schools of Islamic jurisprudence that ensoulment occurs at about 120 days of gestation, after which time abortion is categorically prohibited except to save the life of a pregnant woman. Before that time, opinion differs (Omran, 1992; Mussalam, 1983).

80. See Rosenfield *et al.* (1989) for the proceedings of the 1988 meeting. The International Women's Health Coalition has also sought to redirect the attention of WHO officials towards combating abortion and designing family planning programmes with a greater concern for women's needs (Sen *et al.*, 1994).

81. Charo (1991).

82. See Robey *et al.* (1992); and UN (1998) for overviews of these demographic changes.

83. See Greenslade *et al.* (1993) for a review of MVA clinical and programmatic experience; and Wolf and Benson (1994) on the design of appropriate post-abortion family planning services.

84. See, for example, the edited papers from the second Christopher Tietze International Symposium on the impact of unwanted pregnancy on women's health (Rosenfield *et al.*, 1989); the seminar papers sponsored by the Population Council on abortion research methodologies (Coeytaux *et al.*, 1989); and the papers from a conference on reducing unwanted pregnancy and abortion in Europe through improved family planning services (Newman, 1993).

85. Ford (1991). In time, other foundations also funded a small amount of research in reproductive health.

86. 'Boycott threat forces French company to abandon RU486', *British Medical Journal*, 314: 1150 (19 April 1997).

87. UN (1995b: 61–2). See S. Johnson (1995) for a lively though somewhat partisan account of the conference preparations and proceedings.

88. The phrase comes from Requena-Bichet (1990) who adopts systems theory to describe the interrelationships between abortion as a birth control measure and as a human rights problem.

89. See Cobb and Elder (1972 and 1984); and Kingdon (1995) for discussions of these concepts. Tatalovich and Daynes (1981) applied the agenda-setting approach to the US case, looking at the policy process from the perspective of the life-cycle of the abortion issue.

90. Extensive discussions of elite theory are offered by Putnam (1976); and Bottomore (1993).

91. For studies exploring these cultural dimensions of the US abortion debate, see Luker (1984); and F. Ginsburg (1989). Condit (1990) provides an illuminating exploration of how rhetoric ('the use of language to persuade') has shaped perceptions and policies related to abortion since the early 1960s.

2 Abortion in Kenya: The Tyranny of Silence

1. Widner (1992); and Miller and Yeager (1994). In 1990, for example, the repression of government critics included the 'mysterious' deaths

of Foreign Minister Robert Ouko and Bishop Alexander Muge (from the Church of the Province of Kenya).

2. See, for example, Widner (1992); and Hyden and Bratton (1992).

3. In 1980, 73 per cent of Kenyans were Christians (Barrett, 1982). This proportion is widely thought to have risen since, although accurate estimates are unavailable. Every fourth Christian is believed to be a member of one of the several hundred African independent (indigenous) churches, which broke away from the missions and have continued to separate from each other. For statistics about the Catholic Church in Africa and elsewhere, see Foy and Avato (1996).

4. Interviews with former and present personnel of the KCS Medical Department, Nairobi, December 1991. The Kenya Catholic Secretariat is directed by a secretary general, and a bishop supervises each of its seven departments.

5. See, for example, Radel (1973); and Warwick (1982).

6. See the survey by Cook and Dickens (1981) which remains instructive in this regard. Francophone countries have tended to be even more restrictive on contraception and abortion (Knoppers *et al.*, 1990). Zambia first permitted abortion on broad grounds through the twelfth week of pregnancy in 1973. Botswana, Burundi, Ghana, Seychelles, and Togo had also significantly altered their colonial statutes on abortion (UN, 1992; 1993; and 1995a) before South Africa revised its rules. In practice, the availability of legal services is restricted in all these countries by resource constraints, cumbersome and poorly understood requirements.

7. The text of the 1996 South African law is reprinted in the *International Digest of Health Legislation*, 48 (2): 178–81. No age limit is set, with minors not requiring parental consent to quality for an abortion during the first 12 weeks of pregnancy. Women may terminate their pregnancies for a further eight weeks, subject to broadly defined circumstances.

8. Sections 158, 159 and 160 prohibit attempts to procure, perform or supply dangerous instruments for abortion. Section 228 makes child-killing a felony, whereas section 240 permits abortion to preserve a pregnant woman's life with regard to the patient's state and circumstances. Limited recognition of abortion on broader health grounds, based on the 1938 English *Rex v. Bourne* ruling, is qualified by a more restrictive decision, *Mehar Singh Bansel* v. *R.* (1959), which upheld a charge of manslaughter based on gross negligence against a physician who treated in his office a woman apparently already bleeding from the vagina, presumably after an attempted abortion (Uche, 1974; and Osodo, 1986).

9. Aggarwal and Mati (1980). A similar fate befell hospital reports from other African countries (Liskin, 1980). See Lema and Kabeberi-Macharia (1990) for an annotated bibliography of reports and studies of abortion in Kenya; and Coeytaux (1988) and Rogo (1996) on the demography of abortion in Africa.

10. Interviews with demographers and various health care workers, Nairobi, October–December 1991.

11. Harbison and Robinson (1990). In most populations, total potential fertility (otherwise known as total fecundity) is about 15 births per

woman. In actuality, birth rates are lower due to the fertility-limiting effects of delayed marriage and marital disruption, the use of contraception and induced abortion, and infecundability following childbirth brought about by breastfeeding or abstinence (Bongaarts and Potter, 1983).

12. Mosley *et al.* (1982); and Kalule-Sabiti (1984).
13. Government of Kenya (1989). The proportion of women wanting no more children increases steadily with the number of living children.
14. Kekovole (1991). See also Baker and Khasiani (1992) for case histories of 30 low-income urban women (predominantly adolescents and unmarried women under 25) who underwent induced abortion and in many cases suffered adverse outcomes.
15. Lema *et al.* (1989: 44).
16. See Boerma and Mati (1989); and Ruminjo (1990). The higher estimate is by WHO/UNICEF (1996).
17. Interviews with personnel from Kenyatta National Hospital and IPAS (International Projects Assistance Services), who stated that these figures are more accurate than earlier estimates of over 40 daily cases. Medical professionals point out that incomplete abortions are the major cause of gynaecological admissions at most public hospitals and health centres across Kenya.
18. See Wanjala *et al.* (1985); Murugu (1985); and Aggarwal and Mati (1980; and 1982). Similar findings have been reported elsewhere in Africa (Kinoti *et al.*, 1995; Rogo, 1996). Research and discussion of abortion in Kenya has been dominated by urban hospital-based studies centred on Kenyatta National Hospital's infamous Ward 6, the emergency gynaecological ward attending to incomplete abortions and abortion-related complications.
19. A comparison of two district hospital sites found that the use of MVA instead of D&C reduced the average duration of patient stay by between 49 per cent and 76 per cent, helping lower average patient costs by between 23 per cent and 66 per cent (B.R. Johnson *et al.*, 1992).
20. Lema *et al.* (1989); and for US data, see Lawson *et al.* (1994).
21. See Kelley and Nobbe (1990); Robinson (1992); and Brass and Jolly (1993) on the changes in fertility and family planning behaviour which began in the 1980s.
22. Data from the 1989 and 1993 KDHS surveys. See Ngau and Lema (1988); and Ajayi *et al.* (1991) for studies of adolescent sexual activity in Kenya. The scale of the problems associated with adolescent sexual activity and unwanted pregnancy in Africa is thought to be greater than elsewhere in the world (Bledsoe and Cohen, 1993; and McDevitt *et al.*, 1996).
23. The 1989 KDHS determined the median age at first marriage as 19.8 years for women aged 20–24, compared to 17.3 years for those aged 40–44.
24. A 1985 survey found that fewer than 8 per cent of adolescents aged 12–19 could identify the fertile period in a woman's menstrual cycle (Ajayi *et al.*, 1991), highlighting the need to develop youth counselling facilities. See also Kekovole (1991).

25. Fergusson (1988). Schoolgirls found to be pregnant were usually expelled until a 1994 directive permitted such girls to return to school after giving birth.
26. By way of illustration, as recently as the early 1980s, parenthood was not only a precondition for full adult status, but the middle-aged childless were scorned and driven from their local communities among the Tiriki in Western Province, who are nearly all practising Protestants and functionally literate (Sangree, 1987).
27. Kenyan family life and marriage customs have been undergoing profound transition as a result of rapid socio-economic and ideational changes since at least the mid-1970s (Whiting, 1977; Kuria, 1987; and other essays in Parkin and Nyamwaya, 1987). Men have also become more receptive to the idea of smaller family size, as reflected in the KDHS and other surveys.
28. Cited in Kelley and Nobbe (1990: 20).
29. Interviews with founder and committee members of the Centre for the Study of Adolescence, October–December 1991.
30. Interviews, A. Johnston (Consultant to the NCPD) and J. Kekovole (Chief Demographer, Central Bureau of Statistics), November and December 1991.
31. Baker and Khasiani (1992).
32. As spoken by Archbishop Njenga, then Chairman of the Kenya Episcopal Conference (Njenga, 1980: 5).
33. Kenya Episcopal Conference (1979: 4).
34. Muchai (1985); and Njenga (1985).
35. The Cardinal's statements made front page news ('Otunga hits at birth control', and 'Church backs family planning', *Standard*, 18 and 24 June 1984).
36. The author's interviews with staff members of the KCS and the Family Life Counselling Association of Kenya confirmed that these included the National Right to Life Committee and Human Life International from the USA; the Swiss-based International Right to Life Federation; Women for Life, a group from New Zealand; Women who Want to be Women, a group from Australia; Laissez les Vivres ('Let them Live'), a French group; and Irish Catholic missionary nuns.
37. The two-day meeting, organized as part of the celebrations for the African International Holy Family Year, registered Catholic protests against the proposed agenda of the Cairo conference (as reported in (The *Standard*, 18, 22, 23, 24 and 30 August 1994).
38. As stated in several interviews with the author; and as recorded by Njai (1985); and O'Sullivan (c. 1984).
39. Author's interviews with lawyers (Nairobi, November and December 1991). The Chairman of the Kenya Law Reform Commission had earlier suggested the need to review the law on abortion (ANPPCAN, 1989).
40. This call came at a workshop organized by the Ministry of Health to review the use of MVA (IPAS, 1991; and 'Abortion: Oliech calls for policy guidelines', *Sunday Nation*, 21 July 1991).
41. 'Task force urged to erase abortion laws', *Daily Nation*, 30 October 1991.

42. Interview, D.M. Kiarie (Deputy Director, Family Life Programme, NCCK), December 1991. The NCCK press statement (National Council of Churches of Kenya, 1991) followed less dismissive pronouncements on contraception and sexuality (for example, National Council of Churches of Kenya, 1989).

43. See the reports of the conference by Mbugua *et al.* (1993: 3); and 'Africa's spotlight turns to youth', *Passages*, 11 (3): 8–11 (published by the International Center on Adolescent Fertility, Washington, DC).

44. See Stamp (1991) for an informative discussion of patriarchal and ethnic interpretations of tradition.

45. Kalilombe (1991) observed similar dialectical tendencies in the Catholic Church across Africa. Note that many of Kenya's bishops, including Cardinal Otunga, studied in Rome, while others studied in Ireland, another centre of orthodoxy. Eucharistic congresses are occasions when Catholics celebrate and meditate on the sacrament of communion. They are held about every four years and attended by thousands of Catholics from around the world. Pope John Paul II described the 1985 congress in Nairobi as 'a sign of a new stage of maturity and vigor in the life of the young and thriving church in Africa' (Agunda and Muchiri, 1987: 19).

46. Cited in Okullu (1987: 53).

47. As noted in Kenya Episcopal Conference (1979: 9); Baur (1990: 223); and Okullu (1987: 3 and 53). This is significant because Kenyan presidents have exercised leadership in a moral as well as a political sense, with Jomo Kenyatta often looked on as the spiritual father of the country.

48. The information here is based on interviews with members of the KCS Medical Department, the Family Life Counselling Association of Kenya, the NCCK, and various family planning groups, October–December 1991.

49. In 1994 and 1997, Catholic bishops again led opposition to such a move, aided by some other religious groups and parents ('Sex war: Why parents oppose education plan', *Weekly Review*, 16 December 1994); and 'Moi scuppers sex-education plans in Kenya', *The Lancet*, 350–1152.

50. Both the 1989 and 1993 KDHS surveys showed that less than 1 per cent of all women and of all currently married couples used condoms. The limited clinic and survey data point to high rates of STD infection in the general population, which further fosters a rich culture for post-abortal sepsis. Among pregnant women, syphilis seroactivity rates range from 2.7 to 4.0 per cent (Temmerman *et al.*, 1993). Whereas the Catholic Church rejects condoms categorically, the NCCK approves of condom use within marriage. Both maintain that AIDS can be fought through sexual responsibility.

51. 'Harambee' is a Kiswhali word meaning 'pull together'. It was adopted as a national slogan ('let's unite!') to express a common effort of self-help and spirit for nation-building.

52. Interview, Rev. M.K. Arap Toror (Secretary General, Kenya Episcopal Conference), November 1991.

53. Interviews, Rev. M.K. Arap Toror and A. Kiura (Reproductive Health

Unit, Kenya Medical Research Institute, and Chairman, Family Life Counselling Association of Kenya), November, 1991. See also Kenya Catholic Secretariat (1991).

54. Interview with P. Daino, founder of Maria House and co-founder of IMANI (Incentives from the Marianists to assist the needy to be independent), Nairobi, November 1991.

55. This assessment is based on a number of conversations held with all sides concerned and on the author's own observations when attending one such counselling round. The Caritas nurses are an international association of Catholic nurses. Caritas is a Church charity running nurseries, day-care centres, shelters and medical clinics.

56. Njai (1985: 1). Similar expressions may be found in Njai (1982) and Njenga (1980).

57. Quoted in 'Reporter's notebook: Pope's rhino', *New York Times*, 18 August 1985; and 'Pope hits at abortion', *Standard*, 18 August 1985.

58. As reported in 'To Cairo with an open mind' and 'A whole array of views', *Weekly Review*, 2 and 9 September 1994, respectively.

59. Many have claimed, for instance, that Kenya's population problem is a hoax and women should give birth at all costs. See, for example, O'Sullivan (n.d., *c.*1984).

60. As reported in the unpublished draft conference report provided to the author by the Kenya Catholic Secretariat. Meetings were held beforehand to form a Kenyan 'pro-life association' and prepare a draft constitution (Muchai, 1985: 2–3). PLAN, an acronym for Protect Life in All Nations, is no longer active as an organization. This section has also benefited from interviews and conversations with officials from the Family Life Counselling Association of Kenya, as well as with former and present members of the KCS Medical Department.

61. As recorded in the speech delivered by the Apostolic Pro-Nuncio, C. Faccani, at the Fourth PLAN Congress, 8 July 1995, Nairobi (unpublished typescript made available to the author by the Kenya Catholic Secretariat).

62. The African prelates' main concern was 'inculturation', the attempt to relate Christian church teaching rooted in Eurocentric traditions to Africa's own cultural heritage (see, for example, the reports of the Synod carried in *L'Osservatore Romano* during May 1994; and 'At Vatican, talk is of the harsh realities of Africa', *New York Times*, 1 May 1994). The Synod examined the Church's work in the present-day transformations of Africa, rather like CELAM's Second General Assembly (held in Medellín, 1968) did for Latin America.

63. Interviews, J. Kweri (former director, Family Life Programme, KCS Medical Department), and J. Devane (Manager, Mission for Essential Drugs and Supplies, and former medical secretary, KCS Medical Department), November 1991. The 1989 Catholic directory of Kenya listed nine priests as Opus Dei members, only one of whom was an African national, and an unknown number of lay people (Kenya Catholic Secretariat, 1989).

64. National Council of Churches of Kenya (1991).

65. Interview, K. Erickson (Counsellor, Crisis Pregnancy Ministries),

November 1991. The Christian Action Council, founded in 1975 and the largest Protestant 'pro-life' organization in North America, has extended its activities into Western Europe, Japan and now Africa.

66. This section draws heavily on the author's interviews with women's activists, women prominent in public life, gynaecologists and other physicians, family planning managers, academics and a number of other informed observers.

67. This surfaced, for example, when the local hosts were not readily enabled to coordinate the International Federation for Family Life Promotion congress held in Nairobi in 1989. Both the Kenya Catholic Secretariat and the Family Life Counselling Association of Kenya refuse to provide NFP clients with an informed choice over contraceptive options, whereas the Federation accepts this aid condition, entitling it to receive US government funds (interviews with members of the KCS and the Family Life Counselling Association of Kenya, November and December 1991).

68. In 1994 about 3,000 physicians working in the public sector went on strike demanding the registration of their trade union and better pay. The government successfully waited out the three-month long strike (*British Medical Journal*, 309: 77 and 628).

69. Nzomo (1994), whose primary focus is on the structural impediments to women's empowerment. These are formidable, as is pointed out here, but this does not mean they cannot be penetrated. In the early 1990s, there were three female High Court judges.

70. 'Kenyans do some soul-searching after the rape of 71 schoolgirls', *New York Times*, 28 July 1991; and 'Sexism in Kenya', *Weekly Review*, 9 August 1991. Although the tragedy at this secondary school in Meru province received prominent international attention as well as detailed media coverage in Kenya, the anguished public discussion quickly faded. Evidently, much of the comment that followed the incident fell on deaf ears.

71. Arungu-Olende (1984); and Wamalwa (1991). I am grateful to V.M.M. Kattambo (Principal State Counsel (Research), Kenya Law Reform Commission) for several very insightful conversations on these points.

72. See Wipper (1985); and Nzomo (1994) for further discussion.

73. Quoted in 'Wangari Maathai – the forest queen', *New African Life*, December 1991: 8. The Greenbelt Movement started as a tree-planting project and evolved into an internationally lauded environmental group headed by Wangari Maathai.

74. The author was informed that a proxy for finding out whether a physician is performing abortions in his or her private clinic is whether or not he/she has a second car. Several physicians said that many of their colleagues intentionally refuse to assist patients in public hospitals at the same time as carrying out abortions privately at a fee. The evidence is corroborated by Rogo (1996: 18).

75. I am particularly grateful here to discussions with N.A. Mandara (former Medical Program Officer and Medical Advisor to the Regional Director, IPPF Africa Region, 1982–90), and K.O. Rogo (Senior Lecturer, Obstetrics and Gynecology, University of Nairobi), November and

December 1991. KMA initiated its first major public health project in the mid-1980s, aimed at improving the provision of family planning services by its practitioners.

76. Interview, S.B.O. Ojwang (Vice-Chairman, Kenya Obstetrics and Gynaecological Society), and interviews with council and regular members of the KMA and the Kenya Obstetrics and Gynaecological Society, October–December 1991.

77. As put forth in an interview by A.O. Oyoo (Medical Officer of Health, Nairobi City Commission), December 1991.

78. Interview, F. Manguyu (Chairperson, Kenya Medical Women's Association, and Vice-President for Africa, Medical Women's International Association), November 1991.

79. As stated to the author in an interview with the director of a research programme on women and health, November 1991

80. For more information, see the overview of unsafe abortion and post-abortion family planning in Africa produced by the IPPF Africa Regional Bureau (IPPF, 1996b).

81. Interviews with IPAS officials in both Nairobi and Washington, DC. 1991 and 1993.

82. Interviews with administrators, programme staff, and clinical officers of Marie Stopes Kenya, October–December 1991.

83. See Molnos (1968; and 1972) for discussions of how traditional beliefs and social structure placed a high premium on fertility; and Mbiti (1990) on the religious and mystical links between fertility, lineage and the land. For general reviews of socio-cultural influences on fertility across Africa, see Caldwell and Caldwell (1987; and 1990).

84. For an extended discussion of such an argument, see McFadden (1991).

85. Njai (1985: 5).

86. As stated in an interview with the author by the Secretary of the Kenyan Chapter of the Federation of Women Lawyers, Nairobi, November 1991.

87. Ndeti (1973: 7). For example, abortion in the event of improper sexual circumstances could help avoid social sanctions and restore a woman to her cultural and social milieu. Among the Masai of Narok district, who are still a closely knit and very traditional society, abortion was mostly carried out in the event of untimely sexual relationships, such as when breastfeeding (Lema, 1990).

88. It has been argued that for most of Africa, sexuality did not have centrality in the traditional belief system, unlike reproduction. See, for example, Caldwell *et al.* (1992); and Goody (1976). The obsessive concern with premarital chastity and extramarital fidelity is also a feature of South Asian, Chinese, Middle Eastern and North African societies.

89. See the discussions by Strobel (1984); and Ahlberg (1991).

90. This act also desensitizes women sexually, enhances the probability of a woman's fidelity within marriage, and carries a number of health risks. The deeply rooted tradition, then considered as brutal by the churches as it is now by Western feminists who have renamed it female genital mutilation, nevertheless represented an early part of the anti-colonial struggle (as described by Thiong'o, 1965). President Moi

banned the practice, whose recent resurgence in some areas may be due to a backlash against social change. In 1992, 90 per cent of women in four Kenyan districts had undergone some type of 'circumcision' (reported in *IPPF Open File*, June 1993: 17).

91. Shorter (1974: 72). This was also the case throughout much of sub-Saharan Africa (Hastings, 1973; Chanock, 1985: 150–9; and Parkin and Nyamwaya, 1987). To this day, a church wedding carries less meaning for many couples than does marriage within the community of the clan.

92. The religious community has not been united in its criticism of repression. Some churches left the NCCK rather than be part of any conflict with KANU (Widner, 1992: 190–2). The new evangelistic missions from the southern USA dismissed any political engagement whatsoever (Gifford, 1990). Throup (1995) traces the growth of church criticism of government misrule, especially by bishops from the Church of the Province of Kenya. See also the pastoral letters issued by Catholic bishops (Kenya Episcopal Conference, 1990; and 1994).

93. As indicated by Pope John Paul II to Kenyan bishops in Rome (*L'Osservatore Romano*, 4 May 1994).

94. Barkan (1992). This pattern of personal rule has been marked across Africa (Jackson and Rosberg, 1982; Chabal, 1992).

95. To paraphrase Louis XIV's classic statement: '*L'état? C'est moi!*'

96. Interestingly, the same analysis has been applied to the US abortion issue by Ruth Ginsburg shortly before her nomination as a Supreme Court justice in 1993. A strong supporter of legal access to abortion, she argued that the Supreme Court had ruled too broadly in the *Roe* v. *Wade* decision, thereby putting a halt on a political process that was on its way to giving some degree of approval to more liberal abortion policies (Ginsburg, 1992).

97. Accounts of the deteriorating political, economic and social climate are provided by Miller and Yeager (1994); Widner (1992); and earlier by Thiong'o (1977). Ngugi wa Thiong'o, pushed out of the country for his criticism of the Moi regime, is perhaps Kenya's best-known novelist.

3 Abortion in Mexico: Negotiating a Hidden Reality

1. Whereas punishments are listed for abortions performed for non-therapeutic reasons in all Latin American countries, only Cuba, Barbados and Puerto Rico in the Caribbean, and Belize in Central America, permit abortion on broad social grounds (David and Pick de Weiss, 1992). Nonetheless, across Latin America, 'the harshness of the written statutes is alleviated . . . by their virtual nonenforcement' (Isaacs and Sanhueza, 1975: 39).

2. Paz (1972: ix). Octavio Paz, a Nobel Prize winning author, is widely quoted as an astute analyst of Mexico's formative cultural experiences and attitudinal predispositions.

3. See Stoll (1990); and Martin (1990) on the growth of Protestant evangelical churches in Latin America. In Mexico these churches have won

converts in the south, among Indian groups and along the northern frontier, but hold minimal social and political influence at the national level.

4. Quoted in Eagleson and Scharper (1979: 70).

5. World Bank (1997).

6. Informative discussions about the development and operation of this structure are offered by Bailey (1988); Smith (1991); Brachet-Márquez and Kovacs (1992); Centeno (1994); and R.A. Camp (1996).

7. In his seminal and controversial tract to decipher the Mexican reality, Octavio Paz (1961) draws on the symbol of the mask which has continually figured as a rich historical and cultural metaphor in contemporary social and political life. He explores what lies behind such masks as well as what they express.

8. Articles 329–34 of the Federal District's Penal Code define and prohibit abortion, and set out punishments and attenuating circumstances (Barreda Solórzano, 1991). For a compendium of state laws on abortion, see Tiro Sánchez (1991). The application of abortion laws varies insignificantly between states, despite differences in the letter of the law. For example, Yucatán and Tlaxcala theoretically permit abortion to protect the health of the woman, and Yucatán and Guerrero allow abortion in the event of economic hardship.

9. A review of some six hundred cases brought against women in the Federal District found that only one was sentenced for having committed such an act (González, 1991).

10. Abortifacient herbs are more common in rural areas but are also obtainable in major cities (Pick *et al.*, 1996). Aztec Indians are known to have used native plants as obstetrical and fertility remedies long before the Spanish conquest. The first scientific description of the potential use of the *cihuapahtli* (or *zoapatle*) to induce menses appeared in 1866. For more information about this and other indigenous plants, see Pérez-Palacios and Garza-Flores (1994).

11. For example, Gaslonde (1976) summarized the urban studies sponsored by CELADE (the Latin American Demographic Center) on induced abortion and family planning. These suggested a lifetime average of about one induced abortion per woman.

12. For Latin America as a whole, it is summarized in articles by Viel (1988); David and Pick de Weiss (1992); Paxton *et al.* (1993); and Frejka and Atkin (1996). The reader should be wary, however, of generalizations made for a vast and heterogenous region based on very limited data.

13. By way of illustration, the survey director of the 1987 National Fertility and Health Survey told the author that only 14 per cent of women of childbearing age said they had at least one abortion at some time, and of those women only 13 per cent admitted to an induced abortion. This is significantly less than can be inferred from international studies and considerably understates the problem (interview, Y. Palma, Demographer, CONAPO, July, 1992). See also Nuñez-Fernández and Palma (1991: 7).

14. Ordóñez (1975).

15. Frejka and Atkin (1996).
16. Mendoza (1991).
17. Singh and Wulf (1994).
18. Whereas hospital records from these four countries showed that only 9 per cent of women hospitalized for abortion-related complications acknowledged their abortions, confidential follow-up interviews by midwives indicated that 67 per cent may have had induced abortions (Singh and Wulf, 1993).
19. The reasons why the price for an abortion is thought to have risen in the late 1980s and early 1990s are unclear, but this finding was corroborated by a number of health care providers interviewed by the author. In 1993 the cost of an abortion performed by a gynaecologist in Mexico City amounted to at least several hundred dollars, beyond the reach of many poor people.
20. David and Pick de Weiss (1992) suggested that nulliparous and single women may account for close to half of all abortions, but their sample drew excessively on college-age students and their peers. The present author's interviews with health care providers suggest that most abortions are still procured by women who already have children and are in union.
21. For example, this has been the experience of the Program for Adolescent Mothers, launched in 1988 and institutionalized in a number of maternity hospitals (interview, A. Monroy de Velasco, Director, CORA Guiding Center for Young Adults, July 1992).
22. Atkin and Alatorre-Rico (1991).
23. Romero (1993).
24. A lively personal account of how this took place is given by the lawyer who argued the *Roe v. Wade* case before the US Supreme Court (Weddington, 1992: 11–15 and 32–4).
25. Interviews with senior members of the Division of Maternal and Child Health, IMSS, July 1992, and August 1993. See also Hernández and Mojarro Dávila (1991).
26. WHO/UNICEF (1996). For the results of the earlier study by the Pan American Health Organization, see AbouZahr and Royston (1991).
27. As recorded by the 1976 Mexican Fertility Survey (UN, 1987), the 1987 National Fertility and Health Survey (Palma Cabrera *et al.*, 1989), and the 1995 National Family Planning Survey (CONAPO, 1997).
28. UN (1987).
29. Singh and Wulf (1994). This is from 8 to 20 per cent lower than in five other Latin American countries studied by the authors. However, these calculations are based on a series of assumptions rather than on nationally representative data.
30. Morris *et al.* (1987); and interview with E. Corona (President, Mexican Association for Sexual Education), July 1992. See also Townsend *et al.* (1987).
31. Interviews with senior Latin American regional representatives, Population Council and Ford Foundation, July and August 1992.
32. Lamas (1992a). Similar polls in 1992 and 1994 yielded comparable results.

33. This assessment is widely shared by those interviewed by the author, be they feminists, anti-abortion activists, or academics. I am also grateful to Maria Luisa Tarrés (El Colegio de México) and Claudia Infante Castañeda (National Institute of Public Health, Cuernavaca) for discussing with me their content analyses of newspaper coverage of abortion (interviews, July and August 1992). Tarrés identified four phases in the course of the abortion debate, each characterized by an increased frequency of press articles, and focused on the attitudes and arguments held by different sets of agents (Tarrés *et al.*, 1991). I add a fifth period that centred around the events in Chiapas. Infante Castañeda examined the reporting and use of abortion data (Infante Castañeda, 1988; and Infante Castañeda and Cobos-Pons, 1989).

34. See, in particular, the review by Ordóñez (1975).

35. See the report of the Interdisciplinary Group for the Study of Abortion (CONAPO, 1976).

36. In this sense, the concept of 'voluntary motherhood' differs from the more recent, broader formulation of 'reproductive rights' which now enjoys widespread currency among feminist circles in the industrialized countries and is finding increasing acceptance elsewhere.

37. The work of the Committee on Health and Welfare of the Chamber of Deputies was partly incorporated in a volume of contributions (Leal, 1980) from a smaller, more partisan group of experts that favoured the legalization of abortion.

38. As stated in an address on Mexican population policy delivered in February 1982 (De la Madrid, 1982). In one of the final rallies of Miguel de la Madrid's campaign, a former director of CONAPO called for the decriminalization of abortion and for greater attention to issues concerning women. Her speech did not subsequently appear in the official PRI record of campaign documents (interview, L.M. Leal, Head, National Commission for Women, August 1992).

39. This declaration, published as a full-page advertisement in major national newspapers on 5 April 1989, began with the words *'ninguna mujer aborta por gusto'* ('no woman has an abortion for the heck of it'). Those signing it included well-known politicians from the official party (PRI), the government, opposition figures, feminists, artists and professionals.

40. As discussed in *Proceso*, no. 666 (7 August 1989): 18–22; and, earlier, *Christian Science Monitor*, 12 December 1983.

41. The details are described by Ehrenfeld Lenkiewicz and Cárdenas Elizalda (1992).

42. Interview, Chiapas State Attorney, Tuxtla Gutiérrez, August, 1992. Although the figure cited is improbably high, and reliable data are unavailable, the author's interviews with senior family planning and health personnel confirmed that abortion-related morbidity and mortality rates are higher in Chiapas than in other regions.

43. The precise legal changes are listed in: 'Publicación no. 103-A-91. Adiciones al Codigo Penal para el estado de Chiapas', *Periódico Oficial*, no. 113 (Tuxtla Gutiérrez, Chiapas: Secretaría de Gobierno), pp. 2–10. The state government of Quintana Roo partly lifted restrictions on

abortion in February 1991, but the measure seems to have been quietly forgotten and dispute was much more localized.

44. Interviews with various participants at the meeting, including R. Benítez-Zenteno (National Autonomous University of Mexico, UNAM), August 1992, who made available a copy of the controversial speech he presented that day (5 November 1990).

45. For an account of the significance of this debate written by a widely respected social commentator, see Monsiváis (1991).

46. Infante Castañeda (1988); and Infante Castañeda and Cobos-Pons (1989).

47. Interview, M.C. Alva López (Counsellor, Women's Aid Center, Mexico City), July 1992.

48. Marta Lamas, co-founder and Director, GIRF, and Editor of the journal *Debate Feminista* (Feminist Debate), points to the writings of the German social theorist and political philosopher, Jurgen Habermas, for inspiration on communicating such an alternative position (interview, M. Lamas, July 1992). Many Mexicans heard such views clearly articulated for the first time in a public forum during the aforementioned television debate about the Chiapas reform measure.

49. As recorded by the 1988 Survey on Determinants of Contraceptive Practice, which sampled three regions of the country (Palma Cabrera *et al.*, 1992).

50. Eagleson and Scharper (1979: 73). John Paul II later dedicated a chapel in honour of the Virgin of Guadalupe in the lower level of St Peter's Basílica in Rome.

51. Like the earlier liberal movement ('La Reforma') led by Benito Juárez, who pushed through the disestablishment of the Catholic Church in 1859, the revolutionaries sought to reduce the vast power of the high ecclesiastical hierachies (Loaeza-Lajous, 1990; and Puente, 1992).

52. Existing studies of Mexican elites have focused on university education as a variable for the identification of these privileged groups. See, for example, Smith (1979); and R.A. Camp (1995).

53. Brading (1989); and Loaeza-Lajous (1990). CELAM II, held in 1968 to discuss the meaning of Vatican II for Latin America, concluded that the Church should leave behind its links with existing power structures and that Catholics should work actively towards remedying the continent's chronic social injustices.

54. The bishops voiced their disapproval through lay groups whose objections were easily neutralized. The process underpinning the radical turnaround in Mexico's population policy has still not been satisfactorily explained, although Campbell (1989) shed some light through interviewing several influentials involved.

55. Blancarte (1991; and 1993); and Metz (1992). President Salinas took office after an election many Mexicans believe he won only through fraud. The official computers mysteriously collapsed when he trailed the centre-left populist candidate, Cuauhtémoc Cárdenas, the son of a former PRI president and who was elected Mayor of Mexico City in 1997.

56. As stated by Msgr R. Godinez Flores, Secretary General of the Mexican Episcopal Conference (quoted in 'Mexico restores Vatican ties',

New York Times, 22 September 1992). Pro-Vida has likewise actively opposed anti-AIDS programmes.

57. Interviews with A. López Juárez (Director General, MEXFAM) and G. Rodríguez (Deputy Director, MEXFAM), July 1992; and G. González Juáregui (Pro-Vida state representative, San Luis Potosí), August, 1992. See also the open letter addressed to the state governor and representatives of state family planning programmes by the 'Movement to Help the Potosinian Family' ('Movimiento de Apoyo a la Familia Potosina'), published in the regional newspaper, *El Sol de San Luis*, 4 June 1992; and the interview therein with the State Governor, 15 June 1992.

58. As reported in *El Nacional*, 30 June 1980; and *Uno Más Uno*, 4 July 1980.

59. See the reports in the influential conservative newspaper, *El Heraldo*, 27 July 1984.

60. For further commentary see 'El gobierno Mexicano, indeciso sobre el aborto, ante la Conferencia Internacional de El Cairo' ('The Mexican government is indecisive about abortion before the Cairo conference'), *Proceso*, 25 July 1994, pp. 52–5.

61. Statement issued by Bishop G. Alamilla as a spokesman for the Mexican Episcopate, cited in *Latinamerica Press*, 22 (48): 2 (27 December 1990).

62. The decree, originally published in *El Diario Oficial de la Federación* (25 February 1991), is reprinted in the annex to Serrano Limón (1991). See also the letters sent by the Director of Pro-Vida to President Salinas, dated 13 May 1991, along with 1,530 signatures; and to the President of the National Human Rights Commission, 2 January 1991 (reprinted the same day in *El Heraldo*).

63. Bishop G. Alamilla (auxiliary bishop to the Primate of Mexico), quoted in 'Chiapas abortion law still stalled, but activists keep debate in high gear', *The News*, 3 March 1991.

64. Interview with Bishop N. Rivera (President, Episcopal Commission for the Family), Tehuacán, July 1992.

65. The Archdiocese of Mexico City issued a major position statement on this matter in its 1988 pastoral instruction on morality and sexuality, *Moral y sexualidad* (Mexico City: Sancta Metropolitana Ecclesia Mexicana).

66. Blancarte (1991) presents data on the divergence between Catholic doctrine and actual social practice in general. However, the Church's influence on fertility behaviour has remained largely unexplored by Mexican researchers.

67. This is clear from conversations held with a number of Catholic women and with family planning counsellers in Mexico.

68. The Billings National Center provides instruction in the use of the ovulation method, for which its promotional materials claim a 99 per cent user effectiveness rate (citing out of context a WHO study). By 1992 the Center had representatives in most states. It is affiliated with WOOMB International (the World Organization for the Ovulation Method), an Australian group.

69. Interviews with staff members, Women's Aid Center and Pro-Vida, Mexico City, July 1992; and as reported in the group's newsletter, *Vida-Sí*, 8 (34): 6. Note that adoption is not a common choice in Mexico due to the strong preference for biological parenthood, guilt complexes surrounding adoption and strict adoption laws.
70. Interview with a former director of the IMSS family planning programme Mexico City, July 1992.
71. As stated in 'History of Church in Mexico', *L'Osservatore Romano*, 30 September 1992, pp. 4–6.
72. Interviews with Pro-Vida state representatives from Monterrey, San Luis Potosí and Mexico City, July and August 1992. See also Loaeza-Lajous (1990: 291) on Opus Dei's activities in Mexico.
73. This section draws heavily on the author's interviews with J. Serrano Limón (Director, Pro-Vida), Bishop N. Rivera (President, Episcopal Commission for the Family) and A. Elena Cantú (Pro-Vida state representative, Monterrey), July–August 1992. See also the official accounts of the international congresses (Pro-Vida, 1990; and 1991).
74. Cited in *Excélsior*, 1 April 1990. The Vatican also sent letters of support to both the second international Pro-Vida conference and the first Latin American regional pro-life conference (Pro-Vida, 1991; and 1992).
75. Maceoin (1991); and Comblin (1992: 449).
76. The meeting was called in light of the conclusions of CELAM IV (held in the Dominican Republic, October 1992) and the UN International Year of the Family, designated for 1994 (*L'Osservatore Romano*, 31 March 1993).
77. The murder of Cardinal Posadas Ocampo of Guadalajara remains unsolved, although the government continues to maintain it was a case of mistaken identity in an outburst of drug-related violence.
78. As reported in 'A call for life and the family', *L'Osservatore Romano*, 10 July 1996.
79. Interview, S. Marcos (Head, Catholics for a Free Choice), Cuernavaca, July 1992. See also the group's journal (*Conciencia*), which includes items about other dissenting voices within the Church; and Press Bulletin 04/92 issued by the Archdiocese of Mexico's Department of Social Communication, which speaks of errors in the group's teaching.
80. The author's assessment is based primarily on discussions held with feminist activists and researchers, as well as other academics and well-informed observers. See also Lamas (1992b); and Lamas *et al.* (1995).
81. Feminism has been mostly a force among urban middle-class women, as in many Latin American countries (Jaquette, 1994). The middle class, however, is a very diverse grouping that also contains many women opposed to feminism.
82. Interviews held with the group's founders and personnel, July 1992, and March 1996; and information handouts published by the group GIRE.
83. Mundigo (1996) outlines the critical role played by earlier abortion research in influencing medical opinion in support of family planning across Latin America.

84. As confirmed to the author by members of these organizations in the course of interviews held in Mexico City, June and July 1992.
85. As corroborated in meetings with various family planning officials. Post-abortion contraceptive services are often of poor quality and equated with IUD insertion or sterilization (see also Family Health International, 1997).
86. Such advice carries implications for funding and employment security, and is almost certainly communicated down to managers from a higher level. The Director of CONAPO unexpectedly called off scheduled interviews with the present author on three occasions in August 1992, underscoring a deep political sensitivity to discussing abortion.
87. Nortman *et al.* (1986). In 1987, IMSS provided 38 per cent of all contraceptives used in Mexico (Palma Cabrera *et al.*, 1989).
88. B.R. Johnson *et al.* (1992). MVA requires a shorter patient stay and fewer hospital resources than do other methods of treating incomplete abortion.
89. Tarrés *et al.* (1991). I have also benefited from discussions with several journalists about media coverage of abortion, especially with S. Lovera (Editor, *Doble Jornada*).
90. Lamas (1992b: 9).
91. See the *Guatemala Safe Motherhood Declaration* adopted in Guatemala City by the Central American Safe Motherhood Conference, 31 January 1992.
92. As reflected in the conference declaration, *Safe Motherhood Declaration of Mexico*, proclaimed on 11 February 1993.
93. By law, the president is limited to a six-year presidential term ('sexenio'). The middle years of the sexennial administrative rhythm tend to be the most active period of legislation. The final year is marked by the passage of power to the next president.
94. Sheldin and Hollerbach (1978); and Ingham (1986). This redefinition of abortifacients is less applicable once the foetus becomes more recognizable and the abortion itself more violent.
95. Many commentators have drawn attention to the civic distrust in Mexican political culture. See, for example, Octavio Paz's writings about 'mestizaje'; Craig and Cornelius (1980); and R.A. Camp (1996).
96. The theme that even mutually contradictory truths can be true, including those which are unknown and which otherwise belong to the imaginary realm, is not only pointed out by Mexican writers. It is also evident in the novels of Gabriel García Márquez, as well as other Latin American authors.

4 Abortion in Poland: Peering into Pandora's Box

1. The Pope's remarks in Rome following the parliamentary vote in August 1996 were repeated equally forcefully nine months later during an ardent sermon in Kalisz, Poland (John Paul II, 1997).
2. Bulgaria, Hungary, Czechoslovakia, Romania and Poland all passed laws broadly liberalizing abortion during 1956–57. Yugoslavia enacted permissive legislation in 1960 and 1969; East Germany did so in 1965

and 1972. On the other hand, demographic concerns led to renewed restrictions being placed on abortion in Romania (1966), Bulgaria (1973), and Czechoslovakia and Hungary (in both cases, from 1973 until the late 1980s). Albania kept its restrictive laws until 1990. For further information, see the comparative surveys by Besemeres (1980); David and McIntyre (1981); and Zielińska (1987).

3. The terms East Central Europe, Central Europe, and Eastern Europe are specific to a set of historical and cultural symbols and understandings. For example, the term 'Eastern Europe' was widely used in 'Western' Europe and North America. An ideologically laden concept, it caused much bitterness in Poland and neighbouring countries. By comparison, the term 'East Central Europe' is more ideologically neutral, geographically accurate, accords better with the preferences of the inhabitants of the region, and has recently found widespread acceptance among regional specialists.

4. For statistics on the Catholic Church in Poland, see GUS (1991a).

5. Penal Code, 11 July 1932, articles 231–4. The criminal acts referred to were rape, incest and sexual exploitation. In other circumstances, criminal sanctions were applied against the woman (up to three years' arrest) and those helping her procure an abortion (up to five years' imprisonment).

6. The law, 'On the conditions under which pregnancy termination is allowed', is listed in *Dziennik Ustaw* ('Journal of Laws'), no. 12, item 61, 8 May 1956. Women aged 18 years or under had to obtain the consent of parents or a legal guardian. The instructions issued by the Minister of Health in 1956 and 1959 are spelled out in *Dziennik Ustaw*, no. 13, item 68, 11 May 1956; and in *Dziennik Ustaw*, no. 2, item 15, 13 January 1960. Zielińska (1987; and 1990) provides the most accurate accounts of the historical development of abortion legislation.

7. This ordinance, issued by the Ministry of Health and Social Welfare *(Dziennik Ustaw*, no. 29, item 178, 30 April 1990), repealed the 1959 order.

8. Ministry of Health and Social Welfare Circular, OZN no. 022/90, issued 16 January 1991. At the time, the constitution still guaranteed free health care. The previous allowance of a three-day medical leave after an abortion was also ended.

9. The code, adopted in December 1991, was reprinted in the medical gazette, *Gazeta Lekarska* 1 (14): 11–14.

10. As noted, for example, in 'Polish limits on abortion create a new clandestine movement', *New York Times*, 28 December 1992; and 'Tough abortion law provokes dismay in Poland', *New York Times*, 11 March 1993.

11. 'The law on family planning, protection of the fetus, and the conditions under which pregnancy termination is possible' is published in *Dziennik Ustaw*, no. 17, item 78, 1 March 1993; reprinted in *International Digest of Health Legislation*, 44 (2): 253–5.

12. Parliament of the Republic of Poland (1994).

13. 'Polish code of medical ethics revised', *The Lancet*, 343 (8888): 47.

14. Based on the author's enquiries in Poland during January 1994.

15. The liberal amendments to the 1993 law are published in *Dziennik Ustaw*, no. 139, item 646, 4 December 1996; reprinted in *International Digest of Health Legislation*, 48 (2): 176–178.
16. The text of the ruling by the Constitutional Court is reprinted in *Rzeczpospolita*, 19 June 1997.
17. For a discussion of the relative merits of the various demographic estimates, see Szamotulska (1985). In some urban hospitals, physicians have reported that as many abortions occurred as deliveries.
18. See David and McIntyre (1981); Frejka (1983), and Blayo (1991) for general reviews of the situation in the former 'Eastern Europe'. Abortion statistics were relatively reliable in this region except for Poland, Romania and Yugoslavia. Popov (1991) describes the situation in the regions of the former Soviet Union.
19. Iglicka (1989), based on a calculation employing the framework proposed by Bongaarts (Bongaarts and Potter, 1983) to determine the fertility-reducing impact of the four main proximate determinants of fertility (marriage, contraception, postpartum infecundability and abortion). In computing the index of abortion, Iglicka used a coefficient which assumed a very low level of contraceptive use among married women. More questionably, Iglicka unconditionally accepts a total induced abortion rate for Poland at the highest end of the range of available estimates.
20. Parliament of the Republic of Poland (1994; and 1995).
21. Author's interview with J. Różniatowski (Head, Department of Obstetrics and Gynaecology, Zduńska Wola Hospital), February 1992. This small hospital serves a catchment area of about 62,000 people.
22. As noted by the State Population Commission (Dzienio and Drzewieniecka, 1996).
23. Parliament of the Republic of Poland (1995).
24. See Jóźwiak and Paradysz (1993). A study of married women conducted in 1968 at a Warsaw obstetric clinic showed that the median age of hospital patients was 31.5 years for those undergoing an abortion, compared with 25.4 years for those giving birth (Tucholska-Załuska, 1975).
25. Author's interview with W. Dec (Head, Institute of Obstetrics and Gynaecology, Łódź Medical Academy Hospital), February 1992.
26. GUS (1980). The Family Survey was conducted as part of the World Fertility Survey programme. In Europe comparable proportions of women rely on these less effective methods in Bulgaria, former Yugoslavia, Romania and Albania. Withdrawal and rhythm are often used interchangeably. See Okólski (1983) for a discussion of the difficulties facing Poland's family planning sector in the 1970s and early 1980s.
27. Note, however, that improved access to modern contraceptives in Hungary and East Germany in the 1970s led to reductions in total abortion rates in those countries (Frejka, 1983; Blayo 1991).
28. Kowalska (1993). The household survey consisted of a nationally representative sample of 8,544 men and women aged 18–49 years.
29. Blairman (1991).
30. Although sex education was introduced in many schools in the 1960s,

earlier than in much of the rest of Europe, little if any reference was made to contraception. Even contemporary medical students and nurses receive no education on sexuality and almost none on contraception.

31. As revealed in the author's conversations with members of the Association of Natural Family Planning, Church health workers, and others who have assisted the family planning programme over many years, primarily in Warsaw and Kraków; and as acknowledged in interviews with Catholic physicians and anti-abortion activists.

32. This section has benefited from the author's interviews with staff from the Family Development Association, March 1992. The Society for Conscious Motherhood, formed in 1957, was renamed the Society for Family Planning in 1970, and then the Family Development Association. The operational difficulties faced by the organization over much of this period are described by Kozakiewicz (1986), its former president and past IPPF vice-president.

33. Author's interviews with G. Mrugała (IPPF Programme Officer, Europe Region, 1990–93), March 1992 and January 1994; and W. Nowicka (Executive Director, Federation for Women and Family Planning), January 1994. Several other groups helped form the Federation, including the YWCA (which is linked to Protestant circles), Neutrum (a civil libertarian group), and the Polish Association of Sexologists.

34. Author's interviews with Bishop A. Nossol (Bishop of Opole and Executive Member of the Senior Episcopal Council), February 1992; and Bishop T. Pieronek (Secretary General of the Episcopal Conference), January 1994.

35. Author's interviews with Rev. S. Maślanka and T. Olearczyk (Department of Family Affairs, Archdiocese of Kraków), February 1992.

36. Author's interview with W. Sokoluk, a prominent sexologist, January 1992.

37. This ensured internal cohesion and avoided the risk of being undermined by the regime, as happened elsewhere throughout the Soviet bloc (Ramet, 1990). See Tischner (1987); and Ost (1993) for accounts of Church–state relations.

38. The so-called Round Table meetings involved negotiations between the authorities and the Solidarity opposition, which provided the dynamic to political reform.

39. Wyszyński (1990: 12). The words formed part of the Jasna Góra vows, made by a million pilgrims in a solemn act of national dedication to the Virgin, Queen of Poland, for freedom of the Church and Poland.

40. As stated to the author by priests, professors, and colleagues of the future Pope at the Catholic University of Lublin, in Kraków, and elsewhere.

41. See Wyszyński (1990) for a compilation of these and additional statements made by the episcopate.

42. Kallas (1991). See also the account of the Church's anti-abortion activities from this period provided by Buxakowski (1990). Bishop Buxakowski is Deputy Secretary of the Episcopal Commission for the Family.

43. As described by A. Wojtczak (Deputy Minister of Health) in testimony

before Parliament in 1989, and quoted in 'Abortion issue in Poland splits the opposition', *New York Times*, 29 May 1989.
44. Wasilewska-Trenkner and Witkowski (1985) describe the pronatalist measures taken.
45. Author's interview with M. Kozakiewicz (Sejm Speaker and Deputy, Polish Peasants' Party, 1989–91; until 1993, President, Family Development Association), February 1992.
46. A. Stelmachowski (Minister of Education), cited in *Wprost*, 1 March 1992, p. 5.
47. GUS (1991: 178–83). This survey, conducted by the Central Statistical Office, was better executed than many other surveys on abortion that received far greater publicity from the mass media.
48. Holzer, Roszkiewicz, and Wróblewska (1988).
49. Hord *et al.* (1991); and Zielińska (1993).
50. Hungary's new law and implementation provisions adopted in December 1992 are reprinted in *International Digest of Health Legislation*, 44 (2): 249–53; and 44 (4): 614–15. The old rules were deemed unconstitutional because they were issued by government ministers. For an analysis of the textual strategies used in Hungary's abortion debate, see Gal (1994).
51. The draft law 'On the protection of the conceived child' is set out in Print no. 465, Sejm of the Polish People's Republic (Ninth term, Seventh session), 28 February 1989. The basis of the bill is described by Grześkowiak (1991), one of its main authors.
52. For the text of the 'Senate bill', see Print no. 553, Sejm of the Polish People's Republic, 4 October 1990. I am grateful to Senator W. Piotrowski for making available to me all materials from the proceedings of the Senate committees on Health and Social Policy, Human Rights and Lawful Government, and Legislative Initiatives and Works, as well as other presentations made at this time.
53. Author's interviews with M. Kozakiewicz (House Speaker, Sejm, 1989–91), February 1992; and O. Krzyżanowska (Sejm Deputy Speaker), March 1992.
54. Letter from Archbishop B. Dąbrowski (Secretary General, Polish Episcopal Conference) to Bronisław Geremek (Chairman, Democratic Union), 6 August 1991. This letter was never publicized.
55. Print no. 798, Sejm of the Republic of Poland, Tenth term, 20 March 1991. This bill would have obliged the state to provide modern contraceptives.
56. The revised bill did not permit an abortion if the pregnancy threatened only the health (as opposed to the life) of the woman. See Pawlik (1991) on the deliberations of the Select Committee, which met from January to April 1991.
57. Krynicka, Osiecka, and Sierzputowska (1991). See also the preliminary report from the Sejm's Bureau of Studies and Expertise, dated 9 April 1991.
58. Author's interview with I. Sierakowska (Deputy, Democratic Left Alliance), February 1992.
59. Interview with M. Miśkiewicz (Minister of Health), *Polityka*, 1 February 1992. See also the detailed criticism of the Medical Code of Ethics

made by the Ombudswoman and sent to the Constitutional Tribunal by the Ombudswoman (document no. RP0/92640/91/I/AR, 7 January 1992); the reports in *British Medical Journal*, 304(6820): 137 and (6839): 1399; and *The Lancet*, 339 (8788): 295 and (8803): 1221–2; and 340 (8825): 963–4.

60. As listed in *International Digest of Health Legislation*, cited in note 11.
61. 'Aborcja zakazana' ('Abortion is banned'), *Gazeta Wyborcza*, 8 January 1993; and 'Krok we właściwym kierunku' ('A step in the right direction'), *Tygodnik Powszechny*, 17 January 1993.
62. See 'Kobieta do domu' ('Woman – stay at home'), *Polityka*, 21 March 1992. Minister A. Popowicz (Government Plenipotentiary for Women and Family Affairs, 1991–92) was interviewed by the author on the day of her dismissal from office in February 1992.
63. Author's interview with B. Umińska (Polish Feminist Association), January 1992. This section has also benefited from discussions with a number of other women's group leaders, including several interviews with I. Nowacka (President, Women's League) and with H. Jankowska and M. Księżopolska (Pro Femina). A report by Helsinki Watch (1992) also pointed to the weakness of women's groups and the lack of clear guarantees of equal rights in new legislation. In addition, Fuszara (1991), Hauser, Heyns and Mansbridge (1993), and Jankowska (1994) describe the problems faced by women's activists and their struggle to preserve legal access to abortion services. For a longer-term perspective on the position of women and their political marginalization, see Siemieńska (1991).
64. The medical profession has long been divided in its attitudes to abortion (Wolińska, 1962; and Besemeres, 1980).
65. Author's interview with W. Dec (Head, Institute of Obstetrics and Gynaecology, Łódź Medical Academy Hospital), February 1992; and testimony of M. Szamatowicz (Medical Academy Hospital, Białystok) to the Parliamentary Select Committee on Abortion, March 1991 (unpublished typescript).
66. Author's interview with E. Zielińska (Institute of Law and Administration, University of Warsaw), February 1992. The author reviewed written reports of the meetings and interviewed committee members and expert witnesses called to testify before the committee.
67. See, for example, Buxakowski (1990); and the strident tone of the bishops' pastoral letter on marital love and conceived life, whose focus is on abortion (Polish Episcopal Conference, 1992).
68. As stated by Reverend T. Pieronek (in an interview given to *Tygodnik Powszechny*, 13 January 1991), later appointed Bishop and Secretary General of the Episcopal Conference. Similar statements were made by other churchmen as well as parliamentarians.
69. Interview with Senator W. Piotrowski, main spokesman for the Senate bill, February 1992.
70. Author's interview with Reverend T. Styczeń (Professor of Ethics and Director, Institute of John Paul II, Catholic University of Lublin; and consultant, Pontifical Council for the Family), Lublin, February 1992. Rev. Styczeń holds the professorship once held by the present Pope at the Catholic University of Lublin. See also Styczeń (1991).

71. Senator A. Szczypiorski, a prominent writer, speaking in the Senate and quoted in 'Senatorowie o aborcji' ('Senators on abortion'), *Życie Warszawy*, 2 October 1990.
72. The phrase is linked to the influential writings of T. Boy-Żeleński. During the late 1920s and early 1930s, this noted essayist provoked much comment when he pointed to the health dangers associated with the large number of unsafe, illegal abortions then being performed (Boy-Żeleński, 1992).
73. Author's interview with B. Labuda (Chairwoman, Women's Parliamentary Caucus, and Deputy, Democratic Union), February 1992. The political culture inherited from the communist era did not allow for individual rights, a notion that opposition groups had fought hard to change and that has proved more difficult than expected to inculcate in the democratic era (Kurczewski, 1993).
74. In Romania, the Ceauşescu regime prohibited legal abortion and restricted the availability of modern contraceptives in an effort to increase birth rates. Despite vigorous implementation, such a policy secured only a short-term effect, after which birth rates fell again (Hord *et al.*, 1991).
75. Author's interviews with Senator W. Piotrowski, and J. Łopuszański (Deputy, Christian National Union), February 1992.
76. As illustrated, for example, in the charts posted alongside the anti-abortion displays mounted periodically in many churches. Churchmen (as well as journalists) have occasionally suggested that as many as 825,000 to 1 million abortions are performed per annum (e.g. Meissner, 1991: 88; and Wyszyński, 1990: 193).
77. This section is based on interviews and conversations with anti-abortion activists in Warsaw, Lublin and Kraków. See also Drążkiewicz (1988) for a description of such groups in Warsaw.
78. Author's interview with O. Krzyżanowska (Deputy, Democratic Union, and Sejm Deputy Speaker), March 1992.
79. The IPPF, the major sponsor of the Federation for Women and Family Planning, devotes just over 1 per cent of its entire budget to its European Region (IPPF, 1996a).
80. See, for example, the resolution on abortion passed by the European Parliament, 12 March 1990, and the letter sent by several of its deputies to the Speaker of the Polish Senate, 13 June 1990. Poland has signed the UN Convention on The Elimination of All Forms of Discrimination Against Women and was admitted in 1991 into the Council of Europe, which requires ratification by its members of all European conventions concerning women.
81. 'Polish senate votes to liberalize law restricting abortions', *New York Times*, 2 July 1994; 'Poland keeps tough anti-abortion law', *Washington Post*, 3 September 1994; and 'Poland's strict abortion law survives challenge', *Los Angeles Times*, 3 September 1994.
82. Quoted in 'Primate calls abortion law "a licence to kill"', *The European*, 5–11 September 1996.
83. As stated by the Pope during a mass attended by over 100,000 worshippers (John Paul II, 1997: 99–108).

84. Remarks to a group of Polish pilgrims during a papal audience (3 October 1990) shortly after the Senate approved its draft bill; reprinted in *Tygodnik Powszechny*, 14 October 1990.
85. 'Z dobrą wieścią' (With good news), *Gazeta Wyborcza*, 9–10 January 1993; and *L'Osservatore Romano*, 3 February 1993.
86. As most clearly articulated in the Pope's eleventh encyclical, *Evangelium Vitae*, which deals extensively with abortion (John Paul II, 1995).
87. See, for example, the Pope's fourth encyclical, *Slavorum Apostoli*, which dwells on the common Christian roots of Europeans (John Paul II, 1985).
88. Letters sent to the Speakers of the Senate and the Sejm by the 'Foundation for the Protection of Life in the name of Reverend Jerzy Popiełuszko', dated 12 September 1990. Rev. Popiełuszko was outspoken in his support for the outlawed Solidarity movement and became a symbol of the struggle against communism. He was kidnapped, tortured and killed by security police in 1984.
89. See the statement of the Synod of the Evangelical Reform Church on the draft law to protect the life of the conceived child, reprinted in *Gazeta Wyborcza*, 8 May 1991.
90. Author's interview with Bishop T. Pieronek (Secretary General of the Episcopal Conference); conversations with Archbishop H. Muszyński (President, Polish Episcopal Conference); and Reverend A. Szostek (Deputy President, Catholic University of Lublin, and Deputy Director, Institute of John Paul II, Catholic University of Lublin), January 1994; and other discussions with Church authorities.
91. The Pope made his remarks in Rome to visiting Polish bishops in January 1993 (Sabat-Świdlicka, 1993; and Weigel, 1994).

5   The Global Nature of the Abortion Debate: Realities and Prospects

1. Kenyan attitudes have yet to be accurately measured. Note that in none of the three countries here examined has a reliable study been conducted asking about degree of religiosity and attitude towards abortion.
2. Earlier discussions of population policy found similar results. See, for example, McIntosh (1983).
3. As argued persuasively for the USA by Staggenborg (1991), who offers an informed account of the 'pro-choice' movement there.
4. For a critique of how appeals to rights have become the central means of addressing issues of public morality in the USA, see Glendon (1991). The emphasis on rights is grounded, *inter alia*, in a cultural stress on individualism. Glendon points to France, Germany and Canada as examples of countries where rights are invoked in public discourse with a stronger sense of community.
5. For example, see Luker (1984) and Ginsburg (1989) on the world views and mind-sets of abortion activists in the USA. The analysis by Luker suggests that behind the abortion debate lies a fierce dispute on the role of motherhood in society. Ginsburg challenges the widely shared view that abortion activists represent two ideological extremes. Her

study shows that they share common anxieties faced by women, particularly the perceived devaluation of nurturance. Feminists hold responsible a male-dominated society for this state of affairs; opponents of abortion assume it is a godless society. These concerns are expressed in a rhetoric of female values.

6. Tatalovich and Daynes (1984).

7. Barreda Solórzano (1991) gives this subtitle to his review of Mexican legal provisions on abortion, but does not develop this theme.

8. The editors of a review of abortion politics in Western Europe and the USA concur with this observation, concluding that: 'More than many other issues, abortion has been subject to continuous redefinition' (Lovenduski and Outshoorn, 1986: 3).

9. Catholicism has long played a large part in the popular culture of Latin America. People live under the influence of Catholic moral thought even if they do not subscribe to it. The Mexican church's significance lies primarily in the power of these values, whereas in Central America, as throughout the rest of Latin America, it rests also in the power of ecclesiastical hierarchy.

10. As suggested by Murray (1960: 168) in his discussion of how censorship should be dealt with in a religiously and morally divided society such as the USA. This is an insightful essay written by a prominent Jesuit theologian on the relation between morals and law, and the frequent confusion of these two orders of reality.

11. In 1984 New York Governor Mario Cuomo, a prominent Catholic politician, made a widely cited speech on the need to distinguish morality and legality in a pluralist democracy (reprinted in Jung and Shannon, 1988: 202–16). US Catholic bishops have since drawn back from publicly criticizing Catholic public officials who do not vote on abortion policy in accordance with official Church teaching. This contrasts with the behaviour of a number of senior bishops in the 1984 US presidential election campaign (McBrien, 1987).

12. Sensitive and carefully weighed accounts of church–state relations in the USA are provided by Murray (1960); and McBrien (1987).

13. This is not to say that the hierarchy always favours lay groups. Indeed, many bishops and clergy are wary of any activities operating in the name of the Church outside of their control, on the grounds that such groups may downplay or reinterpret the *magisterium*, or become excessively politicized. An example is the scepticism shown towards Latin American Christian base communities by the Vatican (Hanson, 1987; and Dussel, 1992).

14. See Inglis (1987) on the influence of the Irish Church in public life; and Desiderio (1993) on the situation in the Philippines.

15. The exception to this rule lies in societies where family planning has been coercively imposed, such as in China.

16. For a discussion of these tendencies, see Seidler and Meyer (1989).

17. The report by the Pontifical Academy of Sciences seemingly contradicted official Vatican views. It suggested a birth rate of two children per couple 'to avoid creating the insoluble problems that could arise if we were to renounce our responsibilities to future generations' ('Scientists

associated with Vatican call for population curbs', *New York Times*, 16 June 1994).

18. In 1996 French Catholic bishops issued a report on coping with AIDS that expressed qualified approval for the use of condoms in preventing the spread of the virus during the sex act. The implied justification of condom use rests awkwardly with Vatican opposition to the use of 'artificial' contraceptives, including condoms, in all circumstances ('Condoms tolerated to avoid AIDS, French bishops say', *National Catholic Reporter*, 23 February 1996; 'Church leaders mix condoms and caveats', *National Catholic Reporter*, 15 March 1996).

19. See Coleman (1989) on the organizational imperatives and predicaments facing a Church which seeks to be universal, or what he calls the institutional dynamics of *raison d'église*. This evokes the concept of *raison d'état* which concerns the actions of governments and states.

20. This is also due to the reforms instituted by Vatican II. See Casanova (1994) on the gradual disengagement of Church leaders from direct political activity in democratic countries, particularly on the Spanish and Brazilian cases. As of the mid-1990s, Poland's bishops had only partly withdrawn from political society.

21. Following the 1973 Supreme Court decision legalizing abortion, US Catholic bishops became far more concerned with the state of public morality. In the 1980s they strongly criticized the inequities of capitalist markets and the morality of nuclear weapons policy (McBrien, 1987; and Burns, 1992).

22. The dichotomy between 'conservatives' and 'liberals' has been widely used to describe two conflicting camps within the Church, but the terms are far from precise. Various writers have traced the broad outlines of these internal struggles, which take place largely behind closed doors. See, for example, Hanson (1987); and the more partisan account by Lernoux (1989), with its regional focus on the Americas.

23. See, for example, Ferraro and Hussey (1990). The authors are two former nuns who left their orders after a dispute with the Vatican over abortion.

24. John Paul II (1993). Unlike most encyclicals that are addressed to all Catholics, *Veritatis Splendor* is addressed directly to the Church's bishops. The encyclical reflects the Pope's assessment of Catholic moral theology.

25. The contents of the agenda reflect the 'mobilization of bias' within the political and social system. This concept refers to the use of power for such ends as controlling the relative priority of issues and preventing opposition to entrenched interests from developing (Schattschneider, 1960; and Bachrach and Baratz, 1970).

26. As discussed for Western European nations by Lovenduski and Outshoorn (1986: 2). The authors use the word abstinence rather than avoidance.

27. As implied by the rhetorical question, 'where is the "M" in MCH (maternal child health)?', first provocatively raised by Rosenfield and Maine (1985). This influential article called on international agencies and developing country governments to pay greater attention to addressing maternal mortality.

28. The Norwegian Prime Minister (appointed in 1998 as the director general of the World Health Organization) called for legalization of abortion in all countries, saying that 'morality becomes hypocrisy if it means accepting mothers' suffering or dying in connection with unwanted pregnancies and illegal abortions and unwanted children.' The Pakistani premier based her criticism of abortion on Islamic teaching (S. Johnson, 1995).

29. In South Korea, for example, the sex ratio rose between 1985 and 1990 to 113 males for every 100 females born and climbed rapidly with birth order to a level of 160 to 100 for last-born children in a family of four (Park and Cho, 1995). Sex ratios at birth ordinarily stand at about 105 to 106 boys to 100 girls.

Appendix

1. As outlined by Glaser and Strauss (1967); and Strauss and Corbin (1990). Grounded theory attempts to link qualitative research to the orthodox 'science' model.

2. The different approaches taken by ethnographers are hotly contested among researchers. In formulating my research strategies, I spent more time reflecting on the interpretative process associated with Geertz (1973).

3. See, for example, the works of the social theorists Michel Foucault and Jurgen Habermas (especially Foucault, 1973; and Habermas, 1984). Foucault refers to locally grounded discourses which interpret social reality as 'discursive formations'.

4. See Skolimowski (1994) for an insightful approach to such experiential knowing.

5. Bongaarts and Potter (1983). See Frejka (1983) for an example of the application of this method to estimate abortion incidence.

6. As found, for example, in the USA (Jones and Forrest, 1991). Female respondents who have undergone an abortion where it is illegal and stigmatized may lie as a rational response to intimate and embarrassing questions about such behaviour. They may do so to keep their self-respect or because they are inconvenienced by an outsider's curiosity (Bleek, 1987). Qualitative approaches provide the only means to obtaining reliable information on abortion in such settings.

7. See Dexter (1970) on elite interviewing. See also Spradley (1979) on ethnographic approaches to interviewing; and Patton (1990) on broader aspects of qualitative interviewing which further informed this study.

Bibliography

AbouZahr, C. and E. Royston (eds) (1991) *Maternal Mortality: A Global Factbook* (Geneva: World Health Organization).

Aggarwal, V.P. (1980) 'Obstetric emergency referrals to Kenyatta National Hospital', *East Africa Medical Journal*, 57 (2): 144–9.

Aggarwal, V.P. and J.K.G. Mati (1980) 'Review of abortions at Kenyatta National Hospital, Nairobi', *East African Medical Journal*, 57 (2): 138–43.

Aggarwal, V.P. and J.K.G. Mati (1982) 'Epidemiology of induced abortion in Nairobi, Kenya', *Journal of Obstetrics and Gynaecology of Eastern and Central Africa*, 1 (1): 54–7.

Agunda, K. and M. Muchiri (eds) (1987) *The Eucharist and the Christian Family: The Theme of the 43rd International Eucharistic Congress* (Nairobi: Star Printers).

Ahlberg, B.M. (1991) *Women, Sexuality and the Changing Social Order: The Impact of Government Policies on Reproductive Behavior in Kenya* (Philadelphia: Gordon and Breach).

Ajayi, A.A., L.T. Marangu, J. Miller and J.M. Paxman (1991) 'Adolescent sexuality and fertility in Kenya: a survey of knowledge, perceptions, and practices', *Studies in Family Planning*, 22 (4): 205–16.

ANPPCAN (1989) *The Rights of the Child. Selected Proceedings of a Workshop on the Draft Convention on the Rights of the Child: an African Perspective* (Nairobi: Initiatives, for the African Network for the Prevention and Protection against Child Abuse and Neglect).

Arungu-Olende, R.A. (1984) 'Kenya: not just literacy, but wisdom', in R. Morgan (ed.) *Sisterhood is Global: The International Women's Movement Anthology* (Garden City, NY: Anchor Press/Doubleday), pp. 394–8.

Atkin, L.C. and J. Alatorre-Rico (1991) 'The Psychosocial Meaning of Pregnancy Among Adolescents in Mexico City', paper presented at the 1991 Biennial Meeting of the Society for Research in Child Development, Seattle, 18–20 April.

Bachrach, P. and M. Baratz (1970) *Power and Poverty: Theory and Practice* (New York: Oxford University Press).

Bailey, J.J. (1988) *Governing Mexico: The Statecraft of Crisis Management* (New York: St Martin's Press).

Baker, J. and S. Khasiani (1992) 'Induced abortion in Kenya: case histories', *Studies in Family Planning*, 23 (1): 34–44.

Barkan, J.D. (1992) 'The rise and fall of a governance realm in Kenya', in G. Hyden and M. Bratton (eds), *Governance and Politics in Africa* (London: Lynne Rienner), pp. 167–92.

Barreda (de la) Solórzano, L. (1991) *El delito del aborto: una careta de buena conciencia* ('The crime of abortion: a mask of good conscience') (Mexico City: Miguel Angel Porrúa).

Barrett, D.B. (ed.) (1982) *World Christian Encyclopedia: A Comparative*

Survey of Churches and Religions in the Modern World, A.D. 1900–2000 (New York: Oxford University Press).

Baur, J. (1990) *The Catholic Church in Kenya: A Centenary History* (Nairobi: St Paul Publications).

Besemeres, J.F. (1980) *Socialist Population Politics: The Political Implications of Demographic Trends in the USSR and Eastern Europe* (White Plains, NY: M.E. Sharpe).

Blairman, D. (1991) *Report on a Mission to Poland*, unpublished report prepared by a WHO condom industry consultant for the Ministry of Health, Republic of Poland.

Blancarte, R.J. (1991) *El Poder, Salinismo e Iglesia Católica. Una nueva convivencia?* ('Power, "Salinism" and the Catholic Church. New bedfellows?') (Mexico City: Editorial Grijalbo).

Blancarte, R.J. (1993) 'Recent changes in church–state relations in Mexico: an historical approach', *Journal of Church and State*, 35 (4): 781–805.

Blanchard, D.A. and T.J. Prewitt (1993) *Religious Violence and Abortion: The Gideon Project* (Gainsville, FL: University Press of Florida).

Blane, J. and M. Friedman (1990) *Mexico City Implementation Study*, Population Technical Assistance Project, Occasional Paper no. 5; report prepared for the Office of Population, US Agency for International Development (Washington, DC: Population Technical Assistance Project).

Blayo, C. (1991) 'Les modes de prévention des naissances en Europe de l'Est' ('Methods of birth control in Eastern Europe'), *Population*, 46 (3): 527–46.

Bledsoe, C.H. and B. Cohen (eds) (1993) *Social Dynamics of Adolescent Fertility in Sub-Saharan Africa* (Washington, DC: National Academy Press).

Bleek, W. (1987) 'Lying informants: a fieldwork experience from Ghana', *Population and Development Review*, 13 (2): 314–22.

Boerma, J.T. and J.K.G. Mati (1989) 'Identifying maternal mortality through networking: results from coastal Kenya', *Studies in Family Planning*, 20 (5): 245–53.

Bongaarts, J. (1990) 'The measurement of wanted fertility', *Population and Development Review*, 16 (3): 487–506.

Bongaarts, J. and R.G. Potter (1983) *Fertility, Biology and Behavior: An Analysis of the Proximate Determinants* (New York: Academic Press).

Bottomore, T.B. (1993) *Elites and Society*, 2nd edn (Baltimore: Penguin Books).

Boy-Żeleński, T. (1992) *Dziewice Konsystorskie* ('Consistorian Virgins'). *Piekło Kobiet* ('The Hell of Women') (Poznań: Kantor Wydawniczy SAWW).

Brachet-Márquez, V. and K. Kovacs (1992) 'Explaining sociopolitical change in Latin America: the case of Mexico', *Latin American Research Review*, 27 (3): 91–122.

Brading, D.A. (1989) 'Mexico', in S. Mews (ed.), *Religion in Politics: A World Guide* (Harlow, Essex: Longman), pp. 180–3.

Brass, W. and C.L. Jolly (eds) (1993) *Population Dynamics of Kenya* (Washington, DC: National Academy Press).

Burns, G. (1992) *The Frontiers of Catholicism: The Politics of Ideology in a Liberal World* (Berkeley: University of California Press).

Buxakowski, J. (1990) *O Nowe Spojrzenia na Problemy Ludnościowe w Ustawodawstwie* ('On new conceptions about population problems in the law'), unpublished paper presented as testimony to the Senate Committees on Legal Initiatives and Works, and on Health and Social Policy, Warsaw, 11 April.

Byrnes, T.A. (1991) *Catholic Bishops in American Politics* (Princeton, NJ: Princeton University Press).

Byrnes, T.A. and M.C. Segers (eds) (1992) *The Catholic Church and the Politics of Abortion: A View from the States* (Boulder, CO: Westview).

Caldwell, J.C. and P. Caldwell (1987) 'The cultural context of high fertility in sub-Saharan Africa', *Population and Development Review*, 13 (3): 409–37.

Caldwell, J.C. and P. Caldwell (1990) 'High fertility in Sub-Saharan Africa', *Scientific American*, 252 (5): 118–25.

Caldwell, J.C., P. Caldwell and I.O. Orubuloye (1992) 'The family and sexual networking in sub-Saharan Africa: historical regional differences and present-day implications', *Population Studies*, 46 (3): 385–410.

Callahan, D. (1970) *Abortion: Law, Choice and Morality* (New York: Macmillan).

Callahan, S. and D. Callahan (eds) (1984) *Abortion: Understanding Differences* (New York: Plenum).

Camp, R.A. (1995) *Political Recruitment Across Two Centuries: Mexico, 1884–1991* (Austin, TX: University of Texas Press).

Camp, R.A. (1996) *Politics in Mexico*, 2nd edn (New York: Oxford University Press).

Camp, S.L. (1987) 'The impact of the Mexico City Policy on women and health care in developing countries', *New York University Journal of International Law and Politics*, 20 (1): 35–51.

Camp, S.L. and C.R. Lasher (1989) *International Family Planning Policy – A Chronicle of the Reagan Years* (Washington, DC: Population Crisis Committee).

Campbell, M.M. (1989) *Mexico's Population Policy Reversal 1970–74*, unpublished Masters thesis, Department of Political Science, University of Colorado.

Casanova, J. (1994) *Public Religions in the World* (Chicago: University of Chicago Press).

Centeno, M.A. (1994) *Democracy within Reason: Technocratic Revolution in Mexico* (University Park, PA: Pennsylvania State University Press).

Chabal, P. (1992) *Power in Africa: An Essay in Political Interpretation* (London: Macmillan).

Chałubiński, M. (ed.) (1994) *Polityka i aborcja* ('Politics and Abortion') (Warsaw: Agencja Scholar).

Chanock, M. (1985) *Law, Custom and Social Order: The Colonial Experience in Malawi and Zambia* (Cambridge: Cambridge University Press).

Charo, R.A. (1991) 'A political history of RU-486', in Institute of Medicine, *Biomedical Politics* (Washington, DC: National Academy Press), pp. 43–93.

Chhabra, R. and S.C. Nuna (1994) *Abortion in India: An Overview* (New Delhi: Ford Foundation).

Cobb, R. and C. Elder (1972) *Participation in American Politics: The Dynamics of Agenda-Building* (Baltimore, MD: Johns Hopkins University Press).

Coeytaux, F. (1988) 'Induced abortion in sub-Saharan Africa: what we do and do not know', *Studies in Family Planning*, 19 (3): 186–90.

Coeytaux, F., A. Leonard and E. Royston (eds) (1989) *Methodological Issues in Abortion Research* (New York: Population Council).

Coleman, J.A. (1989) *'Raison d'Église*: Organizational imperatives of the Church in the political order', in J.K. Hadden and A. Shupe (eds), *Secularization and Fundamentalism Reconsidered* (New York: Paragon House), pp. 252–75.

Coleman, J.A. (ed.) (1991) *One Hundred Years of Catholic Social Thought: Celebration and Challenge* (Maryknoll, NY: Orbis).

Coleman, S. (1983) *Family Planning in Japanese Society: Traditional Birth Control in a Modern Urban Culture* (Princeton, NJ: Princeton University Press).

Comblin, J. (1992) 'The Church and defence of human rights', in E. Dussel (ed.) *The Church in Latin America: 1492–1992* (Maryknoll NY: Orbis), pp. 435–54.

CONAPO (1976) *Grupo Interdisciplinario para el Estudio del Aborto en México. Informe Final* ('Interdisciplinary Group for the Study of Abortion. Final Report') (Mexico City: National Population Council).

CONAPO (1997) *Encuestra Nacional de Planificación Familiar* ('National Family Planning Survey') (Mexico City: National Population Council).

Condit, C.M. (1990) *Decoding Abortion Rhetoric: Communicating Social Change* (Champaign, IL: University of Illinois Press).

Congregation for the Doctrine of Faith (1987) *Instruction on the Respect of Human Life in its Origin and on the Dignity of Procreation: Replies to Certain Questions of the Day* (Vatican City: Congregation for the Doctrine of Faith).

Connery, J. (1977) *Abortion and the Development of the Roman Catholic Perspective* (Chicago: Loyola University Press).

Cook, E.A., T.G. Jelen and C. Wilcox (1992) *Between Two Absolutes: Public Opinion and the Politics of Abortion* (Boulder, CO: Westview).

Cook, R.J. (1989) 'Abortion law and policies: challenges and opportunities', in A. Rosenfield *et al.* (eds), pp. 61–87.

Cook, R.J. and B.M. Dickens (1981) 'Abortion laws in African Commonwealth countries', *Journal of African Law*, 25 (2): 60–79.

Craig, A.L. and W.A. Cornelius (1980) 'Political culture in Mexico: continuities and revisionist interpretations', in G.A. Almond and S. Verba (eds) *The Civic Culture Revisited* (Boston: Little, Brown), pp. 325–93.

Crane, B.B. (1994) 'The transnational politics of abortion', in J.L. Finkle and C.A. McIntosh (eds), *The New Politics of Family Planning: Conflict and Consensus in Family Planning* (New York: Oxford University Press), pp. 241–62.

Cremins, R. (1984) 'Family life education: a call to action', *International Review of Natural Family Planning*, 8 (1): 67–75.

Crenin, M.D. and E. Vittinghoff (1994) 'Methotrexate and misoprostol vs misoprostol alone for early abortion: a randomized controlled trial', *Journal of the American Medical Association*, 272 (15): 1190–5.

David, H.P. and R.J. McIntyre (1981) *Reproductive Behavior: Central and Eastern European Experience* (New York: Springer).

David, H.P. and S. Pick de Weiss (1992) 'Abortion in the Americas', in A.R. Omran, J. Unes, J.A. Solis and G. Lopez (eds), *Reproductive Health in the Americas* (Washington, D.C.: Pan American Health Organization), pp. 323–54.

David, H.P., Z. Matejcek, Z. Dytrych and V. Schüller (eds) (1988) *Born Unwanted: Developmental Effects of Denied Abortion* (New York: Springer).

De la Madrid, M. (1982) 'Miguel de la Madrid on population policy in Mexico', *Population and Development Review*, 8 (2): 435–8.

Desiderio, R.S. (1993) *Population Policy and Philippine Politics: Divergent Opinions of Elites on Fertility Control*, unpublished PhD dissertation, Cornell University.

Devereux, G. (1976) *A Study of Abortion in Primitive Societies*, rev. edn (New York: International Universities Press).

Dexter, L.A. (1970) *Elite and Specialized Interviewing* (Evanston, IL: Northwestern University Press).

Diamond, L. and M.F. Plattner (eds) (1993) *The Global Resurgence of Democracy* (Baltimore, MD: Johns Hopkins University Press).

Dixon-Mueller, R. (1993) *Population Policy and Women's Rights Transforming Reproductive Choice* (Westport, CT: Praeger).

Donaldson, P.J. (1990) *Nature Against Us: The United States and the World Population Crisis, 1965–1980* (Chapel Hill, NC: University of North Carolina Press).

Drążkiewicz, J. (1988) *Świadectwo i pomoc. O ruchach antyaborcyjnych w Warszawie* ('Testimony and help: on the anti-abortion movements in Warsaw') (Warsaw: Institute of Sociology, University of Warsaw).

Drążkiewicz, J. (1991) 'Sztuczne poronienia i ruchy antyaborcyjne w Polsce' ('Induced abortion and anti-abortion movements in Poland'), in J. Komorowska (ed.) *Dziecko we współczesnej Polsce* ('The child in contemporary Poland') (Warsaw: Institute of Social Policy, University of Warsaw), vol. 2: 149–94.

Dussel, E. (ed.) (1992) *The Church in Latin America: 1492–1992* (Maryknoll, NY: Orbis).

Dye, T.R. (1987) *Understanding Public Policy*, 6th edn (Englewood Cliffs, NJ: Prentice-Hall).

Dzienio, K. and K. Drzewieniecka (1996) 'Sytuacja demograficzna Polski: raport 1995 Rządowej Komisji Ludnościowej' ('The demographic situation in Poland: the 1995 report of the State Population Commission'), *Studia Demograficzne*, 3 (125): 75–84.

Eagleson, J. and P. Scharper (eds) (1979) *Puebla and Beyond Documentation and Commentary* (Maryknoll, NY: Orbis).

Ehrenfeld Lenkiewicz, N. and R. Cárdenas Elizalda (1992) 'El aborto, análisis conceptual y bibliográfico' ('Abortion, conceptual analysis and bibliography'), unpublished manuscript.

Family Health International (1997) *Postpartum and Postabortion Family*

Planning in Latin America: Interviews with Health Providers, Policy-makers and Women's Advocates in Ecuador, Honduras and Mexico (Research Triangle Park, NC: Family Health International and Pan American Health Organization).

Fergusson, A. (1988) *Schoolgirl Pregnancy in Kenya* (Nairobi: Division of Family Health-GTZ Support Unit, Ministry of Health).

Ferraro, B. and P. Hussey (1990) *No Turning Back: Two Nuns' Battle with the Vatican Over Women's Right to Choose* (New York: Poseidon).

Field, M.J. (1983) *The Comparative Politics of Birth Control: Determinants of Policy Variation and Change in the Developing Nations* (New York: Praeger).

Ford Foundation (1991) *Reproductive Health: A Strategy for the 1990s* (New York: Ford Foundation).

Fortney, J.A. (1981) 'The use of hospital resources to treat incomplete abortions: examples from Latin America', *Public Health Reports*, 96 (6): 574–9.

Foucault, M. (1973) *The Order of Things: An Archaeology of the Human Sciences* (New York: Vintage).

Fox, G.H. (1986) 'American population policy abroad: the Mexico City abortion funding restrictions', *New York University Journal of International Law and Politics*, 18 (2): 609–62.

Foy, A.F. and R.M. Avato (eds) (1996) *1997 Catholic Almanac* (Huntington, IN: Our Sunday Visitor).

Francome, C. (1992) 'Irish women who seek abortions in England', *Family Planning Perspectives*, 24 (6): 265–8.

Frank, O. (1987) 'The demand for fertility control in sub-Saharan Africa', *Studies in Family Planning*, 18 (4): 181–201.

Frank, O. and G. McNicoll (1987) 'An interpretation of fertility and population policy in Kenya', *Population and Development Review*, 13 (2): 209–43.

Frankowski, S.J. and G.F. Cole (eds) (1987) *Abortion and Protection of the Human Fetus: Legal Problems in a Cross-Cultural Perspective* (Dordrecht, Netherlands: Martinus Nijhoff).

Frejka, T. (1983) 'Induced abortion and fertility: a quarter century of experience in Eastern Europe', *Population and Development Review*, 9 (3): 494–520.

Frejka, T. and L.C. Atkin (1996) 'The role of induced abortion in the fertility transition of Latin America', pp. 179–91 in J.M. Guzmán, S. Singh, G. Rodríguez and E.A. Pantelides (eds), *The Fertility Transition in Latin America* (Oxford: Clarendon).

Fuszara, M. (1991) 'Legal regulation of abortion in Poland', *Signs*, 17 (1): 117–28.

Fuszara, M. (1994) 'Debata o aborcji a kształtowanie się sceny politycznej w Polsce po upadku komunizmu' ('The abortion debate and the construction of the political scene in Poland after the fall of communism'), in M. Chałubiński (ed.), *Polityka i aborcja* ('Politics and Abortion') (Warsaw: Agencja Scholar) pp. 52–67.

Gal, S. (1994) 'Gender in the post-socialist transition: the abortion debate in Hungary', *East European Politics and Societies*, 8 (2): 256–86.

Gałkowski, J.W. and J. Gula (eds) (1991) *W imieniu dziecka poczętego* ('In the name of the conceived child'), 2nd edn (Lublin and Rome: Catholic University of Lublin).

Gaslonde, S. (1976) 'Abortion research in Latin America', *Studies in Family Planning*, 7 (8): 211–17.

Geertz, C. (1973) *The Interpretation of Cultures: Selected Essays* (New York: Basic).

Gifford, P. (1990) *Christianity: To Save or Enslave?* (Harare, Zimbabwe: Ecumenical Documentation and Information Centre of Eastern and Southern Africa).

Ginsburg, F. (1989) *Contested Lives: The Abortion Debate in an American Community* (Berkeley, CA: University of California Press).

Ginsburg, R.B. (1992) 'Speaking in a judicial voice', *New York University Law Review*, 67 (6): 1185–209.

Glaser, B.G. and A.L. Strauss (1967) *The Discovery of Grounded Theory: Strategies for Qualitative Research* (Chicago: Aldine).

Glendon, M.A. (1987) *Abortion and Divorce in Western Law* (Cambridge, MA: Harvard University Press).

Glendon, M.A. (1991) *Rights Talk: The Impoverishment of Political Discourse* (New York: Free Press).

Goldscheider, C. and W.D. Mosher (1991) 'Patterns of contraceptive use in the United States: the importance of religious factors', *Studies in Family Planning*, 22 (2): 102–15.

González, L. (1991) *La penalización del aborto en México* ('Punishment of abortion in Mexico'), unpublished research note on a study of legal cases on abortion in the Federal District, prepared for the Mexican Commission for the Defense and Promotion of Human Rights and for the Population Council, Mexico City.

Goody, J. (1976) *Production and Reproduction: A Comparative Study of the Domestic Domain* (Cambridge: Cambridge University Press).

Government of Kenya (1989) *Kenya Demographic and Health Survey 1989* (Nairobi: National Council for Population and Development, Ministry of Home Affairs and National Heritage; and Columbia, MD: Institute for Resource Development/Macro Systems).

Government of Kenya (1994) *Kenya Demographic and Health Survey 1993* (Nairobi: National Council for Population and Development, and Central Bureau of Statistics; and Calverton, MD: Macro International).

Greeley, A.M. (1990) *The Catholic Myth: The Behavior and Beliefs of American Catholics* (New York: Charles Scribner's Sons).

Greenslade, F.C., A.H. Leonard, J. Benson, J. Winkler, and V.L. Henderson (1993) *Manual Vacuum Aspiration: A Summary of Clinical and Programmatic Experience Worldwide* (Carrboro, NC: International Projects Assistance Services).

Grimes, D.A. (1995) 'Sequelae of abortion', in D.T. Baird, D.A. Grimes and P.F.A. Van Look (eds), *Modern Methods of Inducing Abortion* (Oxford: Basil Blackwell), pp. 95–111.

Grześkowiak, A. (1991) 'Uwagi o prawnokarnej ochronie dziecka poczętego na tle propozycji zawartych w projekcie ustawy o prawnej ochronie dziecka poczętego' ('Remarks on the lawful protection of the conceived child with reference to the proposals contained in the draft law on the legal protection of the conceived child'), in Gałkowski and Gula (eds), *W imieniu dziecka poczętego* ('In the name of the conceived child'), 2nd edn (Lublin and Rome: Catholic University of Lublin), pp. 225–42.

Grześkowiak, A. (1992) 'Prawa rodziny w świetle międzynarodowych dokumentów praw czlowieka' ('Family Rights in International Documents'), paper delivered at the IUFO Conference on 'The legal rights of families', Warsaw, 7 March.

GUS (1980) *Dzietność kobiet w Polsce* ('Natality in Poland') (Warsaw: Central Statistical Office).

GUS (1990) *Rocznik Statystyczny Ochrony Zdrowia* ('Statistical yearbook of public health') (Warsaw: Central Statistical Office).

GUS (1991a) *Kosciół Katolicki w Polsce 1918–1990. Rocznik statystyczny* ('The Catholic Church in Poland. A statistical yearbook') (Warsaw: Central Statistical Office and Sociological Institute of Religion).

GUS (1991b) *Sytuacja spoleczno-zawodowa kobiet w 1991 roku* ('The socio-economic situation of women in 1991') (Warsaw: Central Statistical Office).

Habermas, J. (1984) *The Theory of Communicative Action* (Boston: Beacon).

Hanson, E.O. (1987) *The Catholic Church in World Politics* (Princeton, NJ: Princeton University Press).

Harbison, S.F. and W.C. Robinson (1990) 'Components of fertility decline in Kenya: prospects for the future', unpublished paper, Population Council (Nairobi).

Hastings, A. (1973) *Christian Marriage in Africa* (London: SPCK).

Hauser, E., B. Heyns, and J. Mansbridge (1993) 'Feminism in the interstices of politics and culture: Poland in transition', in N. Funk and M. Mueller (eds), *Gender Politics and Post-Communism* (New York: Routledge), pp. 257–73.

Hausknecht, R.U. (1995) 'Methotrexate and misoprostol to terminate early pregnancy', *New England Journal of Medicine*, 333 (9): 537–40.

Helsinki Watch (1992) *Hidden Victims: Women in Post-communist Poland* (Washington, DC: Helsinki Watch).

Helsinki Watch (1993) *Poland: Freedom of Expression Threatened by Curbs on Criticism of Government and Religion* (Washington, DC: Human Rights Watch).

Henshaw, S.K. and E. Morrow (1990) *Induced Abortion: A World Review, 1990 Supplement* (New York: Alan Guttmacher Institute).

Henshaw, S.K. and K. Kost (1996) 'Abortion patients in 1994–1995: characteristics and contraceptive use', *Family Planning Perspectives*, 28 (3): 140–7, and 158.

Henshaw, S.K. and J. van Vort (1994) 'Abortion services in the United States, 1991 and 1992', *Family Planning Perspectives*, 26 (3): 100–6, and 112.

Hernández, D. and O. Mojarro Dávila (1991) *El impacto de las complicaciones del aborto en la muerte materna en el Instituto Mexicana del Seguro Social*, paper presented at the SOMEDE (Mexican Demographic Society) Seminar on 'Socio-demographic aspects of abortion in Mexico', Mexico City, 10 July.

Holy See (1983) *Charter of the Rights of the Family* (Vatican City: Vatican Polyglot).

Holy See (1994) *Catechism of the Catholic Church* (San Francisco: St Ignatius).

Holzer, J.Z., M. Roszkiewicz, and W. Wróblewska (1988) 'Wpływ religii na przerywanie ciąży w Polsce – wyniki badań' ('The influence of religion on induced abortion in Poland – survey results'), *Studia Demograficzne*, 2 (92): 35–57.

Hord, C., H.P. David, F. Donnay and M. Wolf (1991) 'Reproductive health in Romania: reversing the Ceauşescu legacy', *Studies in Family Planning*, 22 (4): 231–40.

Huntington, S.P. (1991) *The Third Wave: Democratization in the Late Twentieth Century* (Norman: University of Oklahoma Press).

Hurst, J. (1989) 'The history of abortion in the Catholic Church: the untold story', *Conscience*, 12 (2): 1–17.

Hyden, G. and M. Bratton (eds) (1992) *Governance and Politics in Africa* (London: Lynne Rienner).

Iglicka, K. (1989) 'Bezpośrednie czynniki płodności' ('The proximate determinants of fertility'), *Studia Demograficzne*, 3 (97): 37–54.

Imber, J.B. (1986) *Abortion and the Private Practice of Medicine* (New Haven, CT: Yale University Press).

Infante Castañeda, C. (1988) 'The data on induced abortion in Mexico: analysis of the statistics published in the newspapers and its implications', paper presented at the 116th meeting of the American Public Health Association, Boston, November.

Infante Castañeda, C. and Y. Cobos-Pons (1989) 'El aborto induicido en cifras: análisis de la difusión de las estadísticas en la prensa' ('Abortion in figures: an analysis of the data reported in the press'), *Salud Pública de México*, 31 (3): 385–93.

Ingham, J.M. (1986) *Mary, Michael and Lucifer. Folk Catholicism in Central Mexico* (Austin, TX: University of Texas).

Inglis, T. (1987) *Moral Monopoly: The Catholic Church in Modern Irish Society* (New York: St Martin's Press).

IPAS (1991) 'Summary of proceedings: Workshop on the management of incomplete abortion in Kenya', 19 July 1991, Duduville, Kenya (unpublished minutes).

IPPF (1996a) *Annual Report 1995–1996* (London: International Planned Parenthood Federation).

IPPF (1996b) *Unsafe Abortion and Post-abortion Family Planning in Africa* (London: International Planned Parenthood Federation).

Isaacs, S.L. and H. Sanhueza (1975) 'Induced abortion in Latin America: the legal perspective', in PAHO, *Epidemiology of Abortion and Practices of Fertility Regulation in Latin America: Selected Reports*, PAHO Scientific Publication no. 306 (Washington, DC: Pan American Health Organization), pp. 39–49.

Jackson, R.H. and C.V. Rosberg (1982) *Personal Rule in Black Africa: Prince, Autocrat, Prophet, Tyrant* (Berkeley, CA: University of California Press).

Jankowska, H. (1994) 'Prawdziwe oblicza "Pro Femina"' ('A true evaluation of "Pro Femina"), in M. Chałubiński (ed.), *W imieniu dziecka poczętego* ('In the name of the conceived child'), 2nd edn (Lublin and Rome: Catholic University of Lublin), pp. 233–243.

Jaquette, J.S. (ed.) (1994) *The Women's Movement in Latin America: Participation and the Transition to Democracy*, 2nd edn (Boulder, CO: Westview).

John Paul II (1981) *Love and Responsibility*, rev. edn (London: Collins).

John Paul II (1985) *Slavorum Apostoli* ('The Apostles of the Slavs') (Washington, DC: US Catholic Conference).

John Paul II (1988) *Sollicitudo Rei Socialis* ('Concern for social matters') (London: Catholic Truth Society).

John Paul II (1991) *Centesimus annus* ('On the hundredth anniversary') (Boston: St Paul Books and Media).

John Paul II (1993) *Veritatis Splendor* ('The splendor of truth') (Boston: St Paul Books and Media).

John Paul II (1995) *Evangelium Vitae* ('The Gospel of Life') (New York: Random House).

John Paul II (1997) *Jan Paweł II w Polsce* ('John Paul II in Poland') (Kraków: Znak).

Johnson, B.R., J. Benson, J. Bradley and A. Rábago Ordoñez (1992) 'Costs and resource utilization for the treatment of incomplete abortion in Kenya and Mexico', *Social Science and Medicine*, 36 (11): 1443–53.

Johnson, B.R., M. Horga and L. Andronache (1993) 'Contraception and abortion in Romania', *Lancet*, 341 (8849): 875–8.

Johnson, S. (1995) *The Politics of Population: The International Conference on Population and Development, Cairo 1994* (London: Earthscan).

Jones, E.F. and J.D. Forrest (1991) 'Use of a supplementary survey of abortion patients to correct contraceptive failure rates for underreporting of abortion', in UN, *Measuring the Dynamics of Contraceptive Use* (New York: United Nations), pp. 139–52.

Jóźwiak, J. and J. Paradysz (1993) 'Demograficzny wymiar aborcji' ('The demographic dimension of abortion'), *Studia Demograficzne*, 1 (111): 31–41.

Judges, D.P. (1993) *Hard Choices, Lost Voices: How the Abortion Conflict has Divided America, Distorted Constitutional Rights, and Damaged the Courts* (Chicago: Ivan R. Dee).

Jung, P. and T. Shannon (eds) (1988) *Abortion and Catholicism: The American Debate* (New York: Crossroad).

Kalilombe, P.A. (1991) 'The effect of the Council on world Catholicism', in A. Hastings (ed.), *Modern Catholicism: Vatican II and After* (New York: Oxford University Press), pp. 310–18.

Kallas, M. (ed.) (1991) *W obronie poczętego* ('In defence of the conceived') (Pelplin, Poland: Wydawnictwo Diecezjalne).

Kalule-Sabiti, I. (1984) 'Bongaarts' proximate determinants of fertility applied to group data from the Kenya Fertility Survey 1977/78', *Journal of Biosocial Science*, 16 (2): 205–18.

Keely, C (1994) 'Limits to papal power: Vatican inaction after Humanae Vitae', in J.L. Finkle and C.A. McIntosh (eds), *The New Politics of Family*

Planning: Conflict and Consensus in Family Planning (New York: Oxford University Press), pp. 220–40.

Kekovole, J. (1991) *Youth Fertility Management Survey: Basic Report Findings and Recommendations* (Nairobi: Family Planning Association of Kenya).

Kelley, A.C. and C.E. Nobbe (1990) *Kenya at the Demographic Turning Point? Hypotheses and a Proposed Research Agenda*, World Bank Discussion Paper, no. 107 (Washington, DC: World Bank).

Kenya Catholic Secretariat (1989) *The Catholic Directory of Kenya* (Nairobi: KCS).

Kenya Catholic Secretariat (1991) *Report on KCS Family Life Program Activities, 1981–February 1991* (Nairobi: KCS Medical Dept).

Kenya Episcopal Conference (1979) *Family and Responsible Parenthood*, pastoral letter, 27 April (Nairobi: Catholic Bishops of Kenya).

Kenya Episcopal Conference (1990) *On the Present Situation in Our Country*, Pastoral letter, 20 June (Nairobi: Catholic Bishops of Kenya) (reprinted in *African Ecclesiastical Review*, 32 (4): 186–92).

Kenya Episcopal Conference (1994) *On the Road to Democracy*, pastoral letter, 12 March (reprinted in *L'Osservatore Romano*, 1 June).

Keown, J. (1988) *Abortion, Doctors and the Law: Some Aspects of the Legal Regulation of Abortion in England from 1803 to 1982* (Cambridge: Cambridge University Press).

Ketting, E. (1993) 'The contraceptive situation in Europe', in K. Newman (ed.) *Progress Postponed: Abortion in Europe in the 1990s* (London: International Planned Parenthood Federation), pp. 7–30.

Kingdon, J.W. (1995) *Agendas, Alternatives and Public Policies*, 2nd edn (New York: HarperCollins).

Kinoti, S.N., L. Gaffkin, J. Benson and L.A. Nicholson (1995) *Monograph on Complications of Unsafe Abortion in Africa* (Arusha, Tanzania: Commonwealth Regional Health Community Secretariat).

Kline, J., Z. Stein and M. Suser (1989) *Conception to Birth: Epidemiology of Prenatal Development* (New York: Oxford University Press).

Knoppers, B.M., I. Brault and E. Sloss (1990) 'Abortion law in Francophone countries', *American Journal of Comparative Law*, 38 (4): 889–922.

Koop, E. (1989) 'The US Surgeon General on the health effects of abortion' (text of Surgeon General C. Everett Koop's letter to President Ronald Reagan), reprinted in *Population and Development Review*, 15 (1): 172–5.

Kowalska, I. (1993) 'Abortion problem against a background of contraceptive attitudes and behaviors', *Studia Demograficzne*, 4 (114): 119–48.

Kozakiewicz, M. (1986) 'History and politics of planned parenthood laws in Poland', in P. Meredith and L. Thomas (eds), *Planned Parenthood in Europe: A Human Rights Perspective* (London: Croom Helm), pp. 197–209.

Krynicka, T., J. Osiecka and E. Sierzputowska (1991) *Wyniki konsultacji społecznej senackiego projektu ustawy o ochronie prawnej dziecka poczętego* (BSE Report, Bureau of Studies and Expertise, Chancellory of the Sejm), 20 June.

Kubicka, L., Z. Matejcek, H.P. David, Z. Dytrych, W.B. Miller and Z. Roth (1995) 'Children from unwanted pregnancies in Prague, Czech

Republic, revisited at age thirty', *Acta Psychiatrica Scandinavica*, 91 (6): 361–9.

Kulczycki, A. (1997) 'Religious systems and abortion: representation and reality', Proceedings of the General Population Conference of the General Population Conference of the International Union for the Scientific Study of Population, Beijing, October, Volume II, pp. 781–801.

Kurczewski, J. (1993) *The Resurrection of Rights in Poland* (New York: Oxford University Press).

Kuria, G.K. (1987) 'The African or customary marriage in Kenya law today', in D. Parkin and D. Nyamwaya (eds), *Transformations of African Marriage* (Manchester: Manchester University Press), pp. 283–306.

LaFleur, W. (1992) *Liquid Life: Abortion and Buddhism in Japan* (Princeton, NJ: Princeton University Press).

Lamas, M. (1992a) 'El aborto en México' ('Abortion in Mexico'), *Nexos*, 15 (176): 51–9.

Lamas, M. (1992b) 'El feminismo méxicano y la lucha por legalizar el aborto' ('Mexican feminism and the struggle to legalize abortion'), unpublished manuscript available from the author and GIRE, Mexico City.

Lamas, M., A. Martínez, M.L. Tarrés and E. Tuñon (1995) 'Building bridges: the growth of popular feminism in Mexico', in A. Basu (ed.), *The Challenge of Local Feminisms: Women's Movements in Global Perspective* (Boulder, CO: Westview), pp. 324–47.

Lawson, H.W., A. Frye, H.K. Atrash, J.C. Smith, H.B. Shulman and M. Ramick (1994) 'Abortion mortality, United States, 1972 through 1987', *American Journal of Obstetrics and Gynecology*, 171 (5): 1365–72.

Leal, L.M. (ed.) (1980) *El problema del aborto en México* ('The problem of abortion in Mexico') (Mexico City: Editorial Porrúa, SA).

Lema, V.M. (1990) 'Abortion: traditional approaches to unwanted pregnancy', unpublished report, Nairobi.

Lema, V.M. and J. Kabeberi-Macharia (1990) *A Review of Abortion in Kenya* (Nairobi: Centre for the Study of Adolescence).

Lema, V.M., R.K. Kamau and K.O. Rogo (1989) *Epidemiology of Abortion in Kenya* (Nairobi: Centre for the Study of Adolescence).

Lernoux, P (1989) *People of God: The Struggle for World Catholicism* (New York: Viking).

Liskin, L.S. (1980) *Complications of Abortion in Developing Countries*, Population Reports, Series F, no 7 (Baltimore, MD: Population Information Program, Johns Hopkins University).

Loaeza-Lajous, S. (1990) 'Continuity and change in the Mexican Catholic Church', in D. Keogh (ed.) *Church and Politics in Latin America* (New York: St Martin's Press), pp. 272–98.

Lovenduski, J. and J. Outshoorn (eds) (1986) *The New Politics of Abortion* (London: Sage).

Luker, C. (1984) *Abortion and the Politics of Motherhood* (Berkeley, CA: University of California Press).

Maceoin, G. (1991) 'Struggle for Latin America's soul quickens', *National Catholic Reporter*, 22 February, pp. 15–19.

Martin, D. (1990) *Tongues of Fire: The Explosion of Protestantism in Latin America* (Oxford: Basil Blackwell).

Mauldin, W.P. (1994) 'Maternal mortality in developing countries: a comparison of rates from two international compendia', *Population and Development Review*, 20 (2): 413–21.

Mbiti, J.S. (1990) *African Religions and Philosophy*, 2nd edn (Portsmouth, NH: Heinemann).

Mbugua, W., P. Kizito, and T. Takona (eds) (1993) 'Adolescent Health in Sub-Saharan Africa: Present and Future', unpublished manuscript, Nairobi.

McBrien, R.P. (1987) *Caesar's Coin* (New York: Macmillan).

McClory, R. (1995) 'Turning Point: The Inside Story of the Papal Birth Control Commission, and how *Humanae Vitae* changed the Life of Patty Crowley and the Future of the Church' (New York: The Crossroad Publishing Company).

McDevitt, T.M., A. Adlakha, T.B. Fowler and V. Harris-Bourne (1996) *Trends in Adolescent Fertility and Contraceptive Use in the Developing World* (Washington, DC: US Bureau of the Census).

McFadden, P. (1991) 'Health as a gender issue', unpublished paper, Nairobi (Centre for African Family Studies).

McIntosh, C.A. (1983) *Population Policy in Western Europe: Responses to Low Fertility in France, Sweden and West Germany* (Armonk, NY: M.E. Sharpe).

McKeegan, M. (1992) *Abortion Politics: Mutiny in the Ranks of the Right* (New York: Free Press).

McLaurin, K.E., C.E. Hord and M. Wolf (1990) 'Health systems' role in abortion care: the need for a pro-active approach', *Issues in Abortion Care 1* (Carrboro, NC: International Projects Assistance Services).

Meissner, K.W. (1991) 'Dyskusja na temat ustawy "antyaborcyjnej"' ('The debate on the "anti-abortion bill"'), *W Drodze*, 9 (217): 82–91.

Melbye, M., J. Wohlfahrt, J.H. Olsen, M. Frisch, T. Westergaard, K. Helweg-Larsen and P.K. Andersen (1997) 'Induced abortion and the risk of breast cancer', *New England Journal of Medicine*, 336: 81–5.

Mendoza, D. (1991) 'Impacto demografico del aborto inducido en Mexico' ('The demographic impact of induced abortion in Mexico') unpublished paper, Division of Reproductive and Maternal/Child Health, IMSS, Mexico City.

Metz, A. (1992) 'Mexican church–state relations under President Carlos Salinas de Gortari', *Journal of Church and State*, 34 (1): 111–30.

Miller, N. and R. Yeager (1994) *Kenya: The Quest for Prosperity*, 2nd edn (Boulder, CO: Westview).

Mohr, J.C. (1978) *Abortion in America: The Origins and Evolution of National Policy* (New York: Oxford University Press).

Molnos, A. (1968) *Attitudes Towards Family Planning in East Africa* (Munich: Weltforum Verlag).

Molnos, A. (1972) *Cultural Source Material for Population Planning in East Africa*, 4 vols (Nairobi: East African Publishing House).

Monsiváis, C. (1991) 'De cómo un día amaneció Pro-Vida con la novedad de vivir en una sociedad laica' ('About one day when Pro-Vida woke up to the news it was living in a lay society'), *Debate Feminista*, 2 (3): 82–8.

Morris, L. *et al.* (1987) *Young Adult Reproductive Health Survey in Two Delegations of Mexico City* (Mexico City: Mexican Academy for Research on Medical Demography).

Mosley, W.H., L. Werner and S. Becker (1982) 'The dynamics of birthspacing and marital fertility in Kenya', *WFS Scientific Report no. 30* (Voorburg, Netherlands: International Statistical Institute).

Muchai, N. (1985) 'Pro-life in Kenya', notes prepared in advance of the PLAN (Protect Life in All Nations) Congress, Nairobi (unpublished typescript, Kenya Catholic Secretariat).

Mundigo, A.I. (1996) 'The role of family planning programmes in the fertility transition in Latin America', in J.M. Guzmán, S. Singh, G. Rodríguez and E.A. Pantelides (eds), *The Fertility Transition in Latin America* (Oxford: Clarendon), pp. 192–210.

Murray, J.C. (1960) *We Hold these Truths: Catholic Reflections on the American Proposition* (New York: Sheed and Ward).

Murugu, N. (1985) 'A ten-year review of mortality due to abortion at Kenyatta National Hospital (1974–83)', M. Med. thesis, University of Nairobi.

Mussalam, B.F. (1983) *Sex and Society in Islam: Birth Control Before the Nineteenth Century* (Cambridge: Cambridge University Press).

National Council of Churches of Kenya (1989) *The Place of Sex in Our Society and the Use of Contraceptives*, press statement, Nairobi, September.

National Council of Churches of Kenya (1991) *The NCCK Speaks on Abolition of Abortion Laws*, draft press statement, Nairobi, December.

Ndeti, K. (1973) *Abortion in Traditional Societies: A Sociological Review of Abortion in Six East African Societies*, paper presented at the IPPF Conference on the Medical and Social Aspects of Abortion in Africa, Accra, Ghana, 13–18 December.

Newman, K. (ed.) (1993) *Progress Postponed: Abortion in Europe in the 1990s* (London: International Planned Parenthood Federation).

Ngau, P.W. and V.M. Lema (1988) *A Review of Research in Adolescent Fertility in Kenya* (Nairobi: Centre for the Study of Adolescence).

Njai, D.M. (1982) *Abortion the Way It Is* (Nairobi: Catholic Bookshop).

Njai, D.M. (1985) *Abortion in Kenya*, unpublished paper presented at PLAN (Pregnant Life for All Nations) conference, Nairobi, 5–8 July.

Njenga, J. (1980) *Religion and Family Planning*, address to the Conference on Population and National Development, Mombasa, 25 August (unpublished typescript, Kenya Catholic Secretariat).

Njenga, J. (1985) 'Family Life Programmes in Kenya', address to the Fourth PLAN (Protect Life in All Nations) Congress, Nairobi, 5 July (unpublished typescript, Kenya Catholic Secretariat).

Noonan, J. (1970) 'An almost absolute value in history', in J. Noonan (ed.) *The Morality of Abortion: Legal and Historical Perspectives* (Cambridge, MA: Harvard University Press), pp. 1–59.

Nortman, D., J. Halvas and A. Rabago (1986) 'A cost-benefit analysis of the Mexican Social Security Administration's family planning program', *Studies in Family Planning*, 17 (1): 1–6.

Nuñez-Fernández, L. and Y. Palma (1991) 'El aborto en México' ('Abortion in Mexico'), *Fem*, 15 (104): 4–15.

Nyong'o, P.A. (1989) 'State and society in Kenya: the disintegration of the nationalist coalitions and the rise of Presidential authoritarianism', *African Affairs*, 88 (351): 229–51.

Nzomo, M. (1994) 'Women in politics and public decision-making', in U. Himmelstrand, K. Kinyanjui and E. Mburugu (eds), *African Perspectives on Development: Controversies, Dilemmas and Openings* (New York: St Martin's Press), pp. 203–17.

Oakley, D. (1977) *The Development of Population Policy in Japan, 1945– 1952, and American Participation*, unpublished PhD dissertation, University of Michigan.

Okagbue, I. (1990) 'Pregnancy termination and the law in Nigeria', *Studies in Family Planning*, 21 (4): 197–208.

Okólski, M. (1983) 'Abortion and contraception in Poland', *Studies in Family Planning*, 14 (11): 263–74.

Okullu, J.H. (1987) *Church and State in Nation Building and Human Development* (Nairobi: Uzima).

Omran, A.R. (1992) *Family Planning in the Legacy of Islam* (New York: Routledge).

Ordóñez, B.R. (1975) 'Induced abortion in Mexico City: summary conclusions from two studies conducted by the Mexican Social Security Institute', in PAHO, *Epidemiology of Abortion and Practices of Fertility Regulation in Latin America: Selected Reports*, PAHO Scientific Publication no. 306 (Washington, DC: Pan American Health Organization), pp. 26–9.

Osodo, M.O.A. (1986) *A Case for the Liberalization of Abortion Law in Kenya*, unpublished LL.B dissertation, University of Nairobi.

Ost, D. (1993) 'Introduction', in A. Michnik (1993) *The Church and the Left* (edited and translated by D. Ost; first published in Polish and French in 1979) (Chicago: University of Chicago Press), pp. 1–28.

O'Sullivan, D. (n.d., c.1984) *Family Planning and Kenya's Future* (Machakos, Kenya: Catholic Mission of Machakos).

Outshoorn, J. (1986) 'The feminist movement and abortion policy in the Netherlands', in D. Dahlerup (ed.), *The New Women's Movement: Feminism and Political Power in Europe and the USA* (London: Sage), pp. 64–84.

Palma Cabrera, Y., J.G. Figueroa Perea, A. Cervantes Carson and C. Echarri Cánovas (1989) *México. Encuesta Nacional Sobre Fecundidad y Salud* ('Mexico: national fertility and health survey') (Mexico City: Ministry of Health, Division of Family Planning; and Columbia, MD: Institute for Resource Development/Macro Systems).

Palma Cabrera, Y., T.J. del Moral and J.L. Palma Cabrera (1992) 'Percepcion del valor de los hijos en tres regiones de México' ('The perception of the value of children in three regions of Mexico'), paper presented at the IUSSP Conference on the Peopling of the Americas, Veracruz, Mexico, May.

Park, C.B. and N.H. Cho (1995) 'Consequences of son preference in a low-fertility society: imbalance of the sex ratio at birth in Korea', *Population and Development Review*, 21 (1): 59–84.

Parkin, D. and D. Nyamwaya (eds) (1987) *Transformations of African Marriage* (Manchester: Manchester University Press).

Parliament of the Republic of Poland (1994) *Sprawozdanie ministrów: edukacji narodowej, pracy i polityki socjalnej, sprawiedliwości, zdrowia i opieki społecznej* ('Report of the Ministers of National Education, Labor and Social Policy, Justice, Health and Social Welfare'), presented to parliament, 21 April (Print no. 375).

Parliament of the Republic of Poland (1995) *Sprawozdanie z realizacji w 1994 roku ustawy z dnia 7 stycznia 1993 roku o planowaniu rodziny, ochronie płodu ludzkiego i warunkach dopuszczalności przerywania ciąży* ('Report on the 1994 implementation of the law of January 7, 1993 on family planning, protection of the fetus, and the conditions under which pregnancy termination is possible'), presented to parliament, 1 December (Print no. 1416).

Patton, M.Q. (1990) *Qualitative Evaluation and Research Methods*, 2nd edn (Newbury Park, CA: Sage).

Paul VI (1968) *Humanae Vitae* ('On human life') (London: Catholic Truth Society).

Pawlik, W. (1991) 'Spór o aborcję, czyli sztuka parlamentarnej erystyki' ('The abortion dispute, or the art of conducting parliamentary argument'), in M. Czyżewski, K. Dunin and A. Piotrowski (eds), *Cudze problemy: o ważności tego, co nieważne* (Warsaw: Ośrodek Badań Społecznych), pp. 123–51.

Paxton, J.M., A. Rizo, L. Brown and J. Benson (1993) 'The clandestine epidemic: the practice of unsafe abortion in Latin America', *Studies in Family Planning*, 24 (4): 205–26.

Paz, O. (1961) *The Labyrinth of Solitude: Life and Thought in Mexico* (New York: Grove).

Paz, O. (1972) *The Other Mexico: A Critique of the Pyramid* (New York: Grove).

Pérez-Palacios, G. and J. Garza-Flores (1994) 'The contributions of Mexican scientists to contraceptive research and development', in P.F.A. Van Look and G. Pérez Palacios (eds), *Contraceptive Research and Development 1984 to 1994: The Road from Mexico City to Cairo and Beyond* (Delhi: Oxford University Press), pp. 233–46.

Petchesky, R.P. (1990) *Abortion and Woman's Choice: The State, Sexuality, and Reproductive Freedom*, rev. edn (Boston, MA: Northeastern University Press).

Petchesky, R.P. and J.A. Weiner (1990) *Global Feminist Perspectives on Reproductive Rights and Reproductive Health* (New York: Women's Studies Program, Hunter College).

Petersen, K.A. (1993) *Abortion Regimes* (Aldershot, UK: Dartmouth).

Pick, S., M. Givaudan, S. Cohen, M. Alvarez and M.E. Collado (1996) 'The role of pharmacists and market herb vendors as abortifacient providers in Mexico City', paper presented at the International Union for the Scientific Study of Population Seminar on Socio-cultural and Political Aspects of Abortion from an Anthropological Perspective, Trivandrum, 25–28 March 1996.

Polish Episcopal Conference (1992) 'O miłości małżeńskiej oraz o prawie wszystkich dzieci poczętych do życia' ('On marital love and on the right to life of all conceived children'), pastoral letter reprinted in *Tygodnik Powszechny*, 12 January.

Popov, A.A. (1991) 'Family planning and induced abortion in the USSR:

basic health and demographic characteristics', *Studies in Family Planning*, 22 (6): 368–77.

Potts, M., P. Diggory and J. Peel (1977) *Abortion* (Cambridge: Cambridge University Press).

Pro-Vida (1990) *Memorias del 1er. Congreso Internacional Pro-Vida. Anticonceptivos: mitos y realidades* ('Memoirs of the First International Pro-Vida Congress. Contraceptives: myths and realities') (Mexico City: Comité Nacional Pro-Vida).

Pro-Vida (1991) *Memorias del II Congreso Internacional Pro-Vida. Aborto: decision de la mujer?* ('Memoirs of the Second International Pro-Vida Congress. Abortion: decision of the woman?') (Mexico City: Comité Nacional Pro-Vida).

Pro-Vida (1992) *1 Encuentro Latinoamericano Pro-Vida, Monterrey, México, 22–24 April, 1992* ('The First Latin American Region Pro-Life Meeting') (Mexico City: Pro-Vida/Pontifical Council for the Family).

Puente, M.A. (1992) 'The Church in Mexico', in E. Dussel (ed.), *The Church in Latin America: 1492–1992* (Maryknoll, NY: Orbis), pp. 217–29.

Putnam, R.D. (1976) *The Comparative Study of Political Elites* (Englewood Cliffs, NJ: Prentice-Hall).

Radel, D. (1973) 'Kenya's population and family planning policy: a challenge to development communication', in T.E. Smith (ed.), *The Politics of Family Planning in the Third World* (London: Allen and Unwin), pp. 67–121.

Ramet, P. (ed.) (1990) *Catholicism and Politics in Communist Societies* (Durham, NC: Duke University Press).

Ranke-Heinemann, U. (1990) *Eunuchs from Heaven: The Catholic Church and Sexuality* (London: Andre Deutsch).

Reese, T.J. (1996) *Inside the Vatican: The Politics and Organization of the Catholic Church* (Cambridge: Harvard University Press).

Requena-Bichet, M. (1970) 'Abortion in Latin America', in R.E. Hall (ed.), *Abortion in a Changing World* (New York: Columbia University Press), vol. 1, pp. 338–52.

Requena-Bichet, M. (1990) 'The problem of induced abortion from the standpoint of human rights', in UN, *Population and Human Rights* (New York: United Nations), pp. 104–31.

Riddle, J.M. (1992) *Contraception and Abortion from the Ancient World to the Renaissance* (Cambridge, MA: Harvard University Press).

Robey, B., S.O. Rutstein, L. Morris and R. Blackburn (1992) *The Reproductive Revolution: New Survey Findings*, Population Reports, Series M, no. 11 (Baltimore, MD: Population Information Program, Johns Hopkins University).

Robinson, W.C. (1992) 'Kenya enters the fertility transition', *Population Studies*, 46 (3): 445–57.

Rogo, K.O. (1991) 'A multidisciplinary approach to policy-oriented research: an example from Kenya', in F.M. Coeytaux *et al.* (eds), *Methodological Issues in Abortion Research* (New York: Population Council), pp. 115–19.

Rogo, K.O. (1996) 'Induced abortion in sub-Saharan Africa', *African Journal of Fertility, Sexuality and Reproductive Health*, 1 (1): 14–25.

Rogo, K.O., R.K. Onango and L.A. Muruli (1987) 'Menarche in African secondary schools in Kenya', *East African Medical Journal*, 64 (11).

Romero, M. (1993) 'Factores de riesgo del aborto en adolescencentes mexicanas: un estudio de casos y controles' ('Risk factors for abortion in Mexican adolescents: a case-control study'), unpublished Masters thesis, National Institute of Public Health, Cuernavaca.

Rosenfield, A. and D. Maine (1985) 'Maternal mortality – a neglected tragedy: where is the M in MCH?', *Lancet*, 8446: 83–5.

Rosenfield, A., M.F. Fathalla, A. Germain and C.L. Indriso (eds) (1989) 'Women's health in the Third World: the impact of unwanted pregnancy', *International Journal of Gynecology and Obstetrics*, Supplement 3.

Royston, E. and S. Armstrong (eds) (1989) *Preventing Maternal Deaths* (Geneva: World Health Organization).

Ruminjo, J.K. (1990) 'Socio-demographic and gynaecological variables of maternal mortality in a Kenyan subdistrict: January 1981 – September 1988', *East African Medical Journal*, 67 (2): 118–25.

Sabat-Świdlicka, A. (1993) 'Church and state in Poland', *RFE/RL Research Report*, 2 (14): 45–53.

Sachdev, P. (ed.) (1988) *International Handbook on Abortion* (New York: Greenwood).

Sander, W. (1992) 'Catholicism and the economics of fertility', *Population Studies*, 46 (3): 477–89.

Sangree, W.H. (1987) 'The childless elderly in Tiriki, Kenya, and Irigwe, Nigeria: a comparative analysis of the relationship between beliefs about childlessness and the social status of the childless elderly', *Journal of Cross-Cultural Gerontology*, 2 (3): 201–23.

Schattschneider, E.E. (1960) *The Semisovereign People: A Realist's View of Democracy in America* (New York: Holt, Rinehart and Winston).

Seidler, J. and K. Meyer (1989) *Conflict and Change in the Catholic Church* (New Brunswick, NJ: Rutgers University Press).

Sen, G., A. Germain, and L.C. Chen (eds) (1994) *Population Policies Reconsidered: Health, Empowerment and Rights* (Cambridge, MA: Harvard University Press).

Serrano Limón, L.F. (1991) *Aborto en México? Crisis o solución? Aniquilar al México joven* ('Abortion in Mexico: crisis or solution? The killing of Mexican youth') (Mexico City: Comité Nacional Pro-Vida).

Sheldin, M.G. and P.E. Hollerbach (1978) 'Modern and traditional fertility regulation in a Mexican community: the process of decision making', *Studies in Family Planning*, 12 (6/7): 278–96.

Shorter, A. (1974) *East African Societies* (Boston: Routledge and Kegan Paul).

Siemieńska, R. (1991) 'Polish women and Polish politics since World War II', *Journal of Women's History*, 3 (1): 108–25.

Singh, S. and D. Wulf (993) 'The likelihood of induced abortion among women hospitalized for abortion complications in four Latin American countries', *International Family Planning Perspectives*, 19 (4): 134–41.

Singh, S. and D. Wulf (1994) 'Estimated levels of induced abortion in six Latin American countries', *International Family Planning Perspectives*, 20 (1): 4–13.

Skolimowski, H. (1994) *The Participatory Mind: A New Theory of the Universe* (London: Penguin).

Smith, P.H. (1979) *Labyrinths of Power: Political Recruitment in Twentieth-Century Mexico* (Princeton, NJ: Princeton University Press).

Smith, P.H. (1991) 'Mexico since 1946: Dynamics of an authoritarian regime', in L. Bethell (ed.), *Mexico Since Independence* (New York: Cambridge University Press), pp. 321–96.

Spradley, J.P. (1979) *The Ethnographic Interview* (Orlando, FL: Harcourt Brace Jovanovich).

Staggenborg, S. (1991) *The Pro-Choice Movement: Organization and Activism in the Abortion Conflict* (New York: Oxford University Press).

Stamp, P. (1991) 'Burying Otieno: the politics of gender and ethnicity in Kenya', *Signs*, 16 (4): 808–45.

Stoll, D. (1990) *Is Latin America Turning Protestant? The Politics of Evangelical Growth* (Berkeley, CA: University of California Press).

Strauss, A.L. and J. Corbin (1990) *Basics of Qualitative Research: Grounded Theory Procedures and Techniques* (Newbury Park, CA: Sage).

Strobel, M. (1984) 'Women in religion and in secular ideology', in M.J. Hay and S. Stichter (eds), *African Women South of the Sahara* (London: Longman), pp. 87–101.

Styczeń, T. (ed.) (1991) *Nienarodzony miarą demokracji* ('The unborn: a test of democracy') (Lublin, Poland: Catholic University of Lublin).

Szamotulska, K.M. (1985) 'W sprawie szacowania liczby sztucznych przerwań ciąży w Polsce w latach 1951–1980' ('The problem of estimating the annual number of induced abortions in Poland'), *Studia Demograficzne*, 4 (82): 105–19.

Szulc, T. (1995) *Pope John Paul II: The Biography* (New York: Scribner).

Tarrés, M.L., G. Hita, and A. Lozana (1991) *Actitudes y estrategias de los diversos agentes sociales y políticos que participan en el debate sobre el aborto en la prensa mexicana 1976–89* ('The attitudes and strategies of social and political agents who have participated in the abortion debate in the Mexican press 1976–1989') (Mexico City: El Colegio de México and the Population Council).

Tarrow, S.G. (1994) *Power in Movement: Social Movements, Collective Action and Politics* (Cambridge: Cambridge University Press).

Tatalovich, R. and B.W. Daynes (1981) *The Politics of Abortion: A Study of Community Conflict in Public Policy-making* (New York: Praeger).

Tatalovich, R. and B.W. Daynes (1984) 'Moral controversies and the policymaking process: Lowi's framework applied to the abortion issue', *Policy Studies Review*, 3 (2): 207–22.

Temmerman, M., F. Mohamedali, and L. Fransen (1993) 'Syphilis prevention in pregnancy: an opportunity to improve reproductive and child health in Kenya', *Health Policy and Planning*, 8 (2): 122–7.

Thiong'o, Ngugi wa (1965) *The River Between* (London: Heinemann).

Thiong'o, Ngugi wa (1977) *Petals of Blood* (London: Heinemann).

Throup, D.W. (1995) '"Render unto Caesar the things that are Caesar's". The politics of Church-State conflict in Kenya, 1978–1990', in H.B. Hansen and M. Twaddle (eds), *Religion and Politics in East Africa: The Period Since Independence* (London: James Currey), pp. 143–76.

Tietze, C. and J. Bongaarts (1976) 'The demographic effect of induced abortion', *Obstetrical and Gynecological Survey*, 31 (10): 699–709.

Tiro Sánchez, A. (1991) *Estudio relativo al delito del aborto en la legislación méxicana* ('A comparative study of the crime of abortion in Mexican legislation'), unpublished compendium, Chiapas.

Tischner, J. (1984) *The Spirit of Solidarity* (San Francisco, CA: Harper and Row).

Tischner, J. (1987) *Marxism and Christianity: The Quarrel and the Dialogue in Poland* (Washington, DC: Georgetown University Press) (translated by M.B. Zaleski and B. Fiore; originally published in 1981 in Polish as *Polski Kształt Dialogu*).

Townsend, J.W. *et al.* (1987) 'Sex education and family planning services for young adults: alternative urban strategies in Mexico', *Studies in Family Planning*, 18 (2): 103–8.

Tucholska-Załuska, H. (1975) 'Przerywanie ciąży ze wskazań społecznych w świetle statystyki szpitalnej' ('Induced abortions performed on social grounds in light of hospital records'), *Studia Demograficzne*, 39: 105–21.

Uche, U.U. (1974) *Law and Population Growth in Kenya* (Boston: Tufts University, Fletcher School of Law and Diplomacy).

UN (1987) *Fertility Behaviour in the Context of Development: Evidence from the World Fertility Survey* (New York: United Nations).

UN (1992) *Abortion Policies: A Global Review. Vol. 1: Afghanistan to France* (New York: United Nations).

UN (1993) *Abortion Policies: A Global Review. Vol. 2: Gabon to Norway* (New York: United Nations).

UN (1995a) *Abortion Policies: A Global Review. Vol. 3: Oman to Zimbabwe* (New York: United Nations).

UN (1995b) *Population and Development: Programme of Action Adopted at the International Conference on Population and Development* (Cairo, 5–13 September 1994) (New York: United Nations).

UN (1998) *World Population Monitoring 1996: Selected Aspects of Reproductive Rights and Reproductive Health* (New York: United Nations).

UN (forthcoming) *World Population Prospects: The 1996 Revision* (New York: United Nations).

UNDP (1997) *Human Development Report 1997* (New York: Oxford University Press).

Vallier, I. (1972) 'The Roman Catholic Church: a transnational actor', in R.O. Keohane and J.S. Nye (eds), *Transnational Relations and World Politics* (Cambridge, MA: Harvard University Press), pp. 129–52.

Van Look, P.F.A. and H. von Hertzen (1994) 'Post-ovulatory methods of Fertility Regulation: the emergence of antiprogestogens', in P.F.A. Van Look and G. Pérez-Palacios (eds), *Contraceptive Research and Development 1984 to 1994: The Road from Mexico City to Cairo and Beyond* (Delhi: Oxford University Press), pp. 151–201.

Viel, B.V. (1988) 'Latin America', in P. Sachdev (ed.), *International Handbook on Abortion* (New York: Greenwood), pp. 317–32.

Walsh, M.J. (1989) *The Secret World of Opus Dei* (London: Grafton).

Wamalwa, B. (1991) 'Limits of women's groups as a viable channel for the development of women in Kenya', in T. Wallace and C. March (eds), *Changing Perceptions: Writings on Gender and Development* (Oxford: Oxfam), pp. 245–52.

Wanjala, S., N.M. Murugu and J.K.G. Mati (1985) 'Mortality due to abortion at Kenyatta National Hospital, 1974–1983', in Ciba Foundation, *Abortion: Medical Progress and Social Implications* (London: Pitman), pp. 41–8.

Warwick, D.P. (1982) *Bitter Pills: Population Policies and their Implementation in Eight Developing Countries* (Cambridge: Cambridge University Press).

Wasilewska-Trenkner, H. and J. Witkowski (1985) 'O polityce ludnościowej w Polsce' ('On population policy'), *Studia Demograficzne*, 4 (82): 33–50.

Weddington, S.R. (1992) *A Question of Choice* (New York: Putnam).

Weigel, G. (1992) *The Final Revolution* (New York: Oxford University Press).

Weigel, G. (1994) 'The great Polish experiment', *Commentary*, 97 (2): 37–42.

Whiting, B.B. (1977) 'Changing lifestyles in Kenya', *Daedalus*, 106 (2): 211–25.

WHO (1992) *The Prevention and Management of Unsafe Abortion*, Report of a Technical Working Group (Geneva: WHO).

WHO (1994) *Abortion: A Tabulation of Available Data on the Frequency and Mortality of Unsafe Abortion*: 2nd edn (Geneva: World Health Organization).

WHO/UNICEF (1996) *Revised 1990 Estimates of Maternal Mortality: A New Approach by WHO and UNICEF* (Geneva: World Health Organization).

Widner, J.A. (1992) *The Rise of a Party-State in Kenya: From 'Harambee!' to 'Nyayo!'* (Berkeley, CA: University of California Press).

Williams, O.F. and J.W. Houck (eds) (1993) *Catholic Social Thought and the New World Order: Building on One Hundred Years* (Notre Dame, ID: University of Notre Dame Press).

Wipper, A.S. (1985) 'The Maendeleo Ya Wanawake organization: the cooptation of leadership', *African Studies Review*, 18 (3): 99–119.

Wolf, M. and J. Benson (1994) 'Meeting women's needs for post-abortion family planning', Report of a Bellagio Technical Working Group, Bellagio, Italy, February 1–5, *International Journal of Gynecology and Obstetrics*, Supplement to Volume 45.

Wolińska, H. (1962) *Przerwanie ciąży w świetle prawa karnego* ('Abortion in the light of criminal law') (Warsaw: Państwowe Wydawnictwo Naukowe).

World Bank (1997) *World Development Report 1997* (New York: Oxford University Press).

Wyszyński, S. (1990) *W obronie życia nienarodzonych* ('In defense of the life of the unborn') (Warsaw: Instytut Prymasowski Ślubów Narodu).

Zielińska, E. (1987) 'European socialist countries', in S.J. Frankowski and G.F. Cole (eds), *Abortion and Protection of the Human Fetus* (Dordrecht, Netherlands: Martinus Nijhoff), pp. 241–334.

Zielińska, E. (1990) *Przerywanie ciąży. Warunki legalności w Polsce i na świecie* ('Abortion: conditions for its legality in Poland and the world') (Warsaw: Wydawnictwo Prawnicze).

Zielińska, E. (1993) 'Recent trends in abortion legislation in Eastern Europe, with particular reference to Poland', *Criminal Law Forum*, 4 (1): 47–93.

Name/Author Index

Subject Index